Basic Questions on

Healthcare

What Should Good Care Include?

T0256067

The BioBasics Series provides insightful and practical answers to many of today's pressing bioethical questions. Advances in medical technology have resulted in longer and healthier lives, but they have also produced interventions and procedures that call for serious ethical evaluation. What we can do is not necessarily what we should do. This series is designed to instill in each reader an uncompromising respect for human life that will serve as a compass through a maze of challenging questions.

This series is a project of The Center for Bioethics and Human Dignity, an international organization located just north of Chicago, Illinois, in the United States of America. The Center endeavors to bring Christian perspectives to bear on today's many difficult bioethical challenges. It develops book, audio, and video series; presents numerous conferences in different parts of the world; and offers a variety of other printed and computer-based resources. Through its membership program, the Center provides worldwide resources on bioethical matters. Members receive the Center's international journal, *Ethics and Medicine,* the Center's newsletter, *Dignity,* the CBHD Internet News Service (weekly and monthly), special notification of Center conferences and publications, discounts on all Center conferences and resources, and more.

For more information on membership in the Center or its various resources, including present or future books in the BioBasics Series, contact the Center at:

The Center for Bioethics and Human Dignity
2065 Half Day Road
Bannockburn, IL 60015 USA
Phone: (847) 317-8180 Fax: (847) 317-8101
E-mail: info@cbhd.org

Information and ordering is also available through the Center's World Wide Web site on the Internet: http://www.cbhd.org.

BioBasics Series

Basic Questions on

Healthcare

What Should Good Care Include?

Dónal P. O'Mathúna, Ph.D.
Samuel D. Hensley, M.D.
Mary B. Adam, M.D.
John F. Kilner, Ph.D.
Robert D. Orr, M.D.
Gary P. Stewart, D.Min.

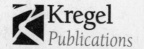
Kregel
Publications

Basic Questions on Healthcare: What Should Good Care Include?

© 2004 by The Center for Bioethics and Human Dignity

Published by Kregel Publications, a division of Kregel, Inc., P.O. Box 2607, Grand Rapids, MI 49501.

All rights reserved. No part of this book may be reproduced, stored in a retrieval system, or transmitted in any form or by any means—electronic, mechanical, photocopy, recording, or otherwise—without written permission of the publisher, except for brief quotations in printed reviews.

Unless otherwise indicated, Scripture quotations are from the *Holy Bible: New International Version*®. Copyright © 1973, 1978, 1984 by International Bible Society. Used by permission of Zondervan Publishing House. All rights reserved.

Scripture quotations marked NASB are from the *New American Standard Bible,* © the Lockman Foundation 1960, 1962, 1963, 1968, 1971, 1972, 1973, 1975, 1977.

ISBN 0-8254-3081-x

Printed in the United States of America

1 2 3 4 5 / 08 07 06 05 04

Table of Contents

Ethics Controversies

Access to Healthcare

Financing Healthcare

Contributors

Mary B. Adam, M.D., is a pediatrician who has a National Institutes of Health joint appointment in the Department of Pediatrics and Surgery. She is also a Fellow of The Center for Bioethics and Human Dignity, Bannockburn, Illinois.

Samuel D. Hensley, M.D., is a surgical pathologist in the Department of Anatomic Pathology at Mississippi Baptist Medical Center in Jackson, Mississippi. He is also an Assistant Clinical Professor at the University of Mississippi School of Medicine and a Fellow of The Center for Bioethics and Human Dignity.

John F. Kilner, Ph.D., is President of The Center for Bioethics and Human Dignity, Bannockburn, Illinois.

Dónal P. O'Mathúna, Ph.D., is Professor of Bioethics and Chemistry at Mount Carmel College of Nursing in Columbus, Ohio. He is also a Fellow of The Center for Bioethics and Human Dignity.

Robert D. Orr, M.D., is Director of Ethics at Fletcher Allen Healthcare, University of Vermont College of Medicine. He is also Director of Clinical Ethics at The Center for Bioethics and Human Dignity.

Gary P. Stewart, D.Min., is a military chaplain serving with the U.S. Marine Corps.

The Center for Bioethics and Human Dignity wishes to extend its special gratitude to Robert Cranston, M.D. for authoring the "Ethics Controversies" section of this booklet. Dr. Cranston is an Attending Physician and Head of the Division of Neurology at Carle Clinic and Carle Foundation Hospital in Urbana, Illinois. He is also a CBHD Fellow.

We wish also to thank Dan Beals, M.D. for his review of this section. Dr. Beals is an Associate Professor of surgery and pediatrics at the University of Kentucky. He is also a CBHD Fellow.

Introduction

Times have changed since simpler days when one general doctor treated every family member from newborns to elderly parents regardless of the medical situation. This physician delivered babies, set broken arms, diagnosed disease, and dispensed sage advice—likely from the same ethical and religious perspective as that of the patient. Today's medical environment is increasingly complex and diverse. Because specialists have replaced generalists and society is increasingly mobile, your primary physician can change often over the course of a lifetime, requiring an ongoing selection process. Unless you are careful, you may well end up with a physician and other caregivers who do not share your ethical and religious convictions. In that case, your need to be informed about the challenges and choices facing you is all the greater.

Healthcare is an arena where the decisions you make will have a radical effect on your life and the lives of your loved ones. To make good decisions, you need resources. You need access to good healthcare, which can be extremely expensive today. You need access to good information, which can be confusingly abundant today. You need access to good communication, counsel, and support—and knowing what to expect regarding these and how to obtain what you need can be extraordinarily difficult.

This book is designed to give you the understanding and biblical perspective necessary so that you can truly experience healthcare today as a form of care and a means of health. While answers to particular questions will provide

11

you targeted information for specific needs, you will find that reading the book through as a whole now will help you be ready when healthcare challenges inevitably arise in the days ahead.

This book is not intended to reproduce all the available information on the subjects addressed but rather to simplify, complement, and supplement other available resources that the reader is encouraged to consult. (Some of these materials have been listed at the end of this book.) This book is not intended to take the place of theological, legal, medical, or psychological counsel or treatment. If assistance in any of these areas is needed, please seek the services of a certified professional. The views expressed in this work are solely those of the authors and do not represent or reflect the position or endorsement of any governmental agency or department, military or otherwise.

1. What is the Hippocratic Oath?

In answering this question, it is important to review briefly not only the Oath's content, but also its history and the culture in which it originated.[1] Such a review is important in understanding the demands that the Oath places on contemporary physicians.

Although many of the historical details have been lost over time, it's clear that the Oath first originated in ancient Greece between 600 and 400 B.C. and came to be associated with Hippocrates of Cos, who was himself a physician. It is significant that the ideals embodied in the Oath were contrary to general medical practice in ancient Greece and the surrounding cultures, where abortion and physician-assisted suicide were commonly practiced and regarded as socially acceptable. Physicians in the time of Hippocrates were allowed either to attempt to heal patients or to administer a fatal poison to end their suffering. With few effective treatments to relieve pain, physicians were often asked to administer poison, and they often willingly complied. Abortion was also frequent, given the promiscuous lifestyles and lack of birth control. From antiquity, religious figures such as priests or other representatives of the pagan religious establishment have been closely connected to the art of healing. The primary reason for this association was that illness was often considered to be a consequence of having offended one of the gods. It's not surprising, then, that religious figures were (and are) often involved in healing.

The contents of the Hippocratic Oath were revolutionary in many ways. Three particularly important aspects of the Oath follow:

1. *Medicine as a moral enterprise.* Medical education in the time of Hippocrates began with students in the Hippocratic School swearing the Oath by the "gods." Such a practice reflected the understanding that treating the sick and attending to the suffering are moral acts. Medicine is more than mere technique—it is technique inseparably bonded to certain moral commitments expressed in the Oath. Christianity also affirms that caring for patients has an inherent moral dimension since it is done before the face of God.

2. *Sanctity of life.* Although the term "sanctity of life" is not present in the Oath, the principle is, nevertheless, apparent in that the Oath forbids the physician to kill. Students taking the Oath swore never to administer poison to a patient even if the patient requested it (physician-assisted suicide) or to give a woman a pessary to induce an abortion. The Bible similarly upholds the value of all human life because it carries the image of God.

3. *Covenant.* Upon taking the Oath, the Hippocratic physician-in-training was placed in a complex covenantal relationship, pledging responsibility to his teacher, to his patients, and to the gods. This threefold covenant and its underlying moral commitments served to shape the practice of medicine. For contemporary Christian physicians, the Hippocratic Oath is not viewed as a simple code of ethics; rather, it's regarded as a covenant with God that shapes and defines all aspects of the physician/patient relationship.

In the time of Hippocrates, Greek religion was polytheistic—being rooted in a whole pantheon of gods. These early Greeks were not aware of the God of Abraham,

Isaac, and Jacob. Still, through God's common grace, Hippocrates concluded that human life was sacred and that physicians should strive to promote human flourishing and well-being. Hippocrates declared that human life was sacred because the gods had created it. When Christians encountered the Oath centuries later, they realized it was an eloquent statement embodying biblical truth and, therefore, they easily adapted it for their own use. (The full text of the Oath is provided in the appendix.)

2. Is the Hippocratic Oath still the standard of good medical practice?

The importance of the Hippocratic Oath and its role in shaping the standards of medical practice for the past twenty-four hundred years cannot be overemphasized. As stated in the previous answer, the Oath affirms the moral nature of medicine and promotes high moral standards. Not only does the Oath reject the killing of patients, it calls on physicians to live pure and holy lives. It addresses issues of justice, money, and confidentiality and offers counsel on relationships with patients and colleagues. As such, the Oath's guiding principles remain the standard of good medical practice.

Although the Hippocratic Oath formed the basis for the practice of medicine and guided it for over two thousand years, it has been under unrelenting attack in recent years. In the late twentieth century, many cultural characteristics of pre-Hippocratic paganism recurred, especially in Western Europe and the United States. The perceived acceptability—and even desirability—of allowing physicians to kill their patients has steadily increased. With this trend toward physician-assisted suicide and the legally recognized "right" of women to choose abortion, the Hippocratic mandate that physicians should heal—and not harm—their patients has been seriously challenged. Although the decline in Hippocratic medicine is disturbing, individual physicians are not precluded from remaining faithful to Hippocratic precepts. Indeed, the original Hippocratic physicians flourished despite living in a predominantly pagan society.

Hippocratic medicine continues to be practiced and must remain a defining feature of Christian physicians.[2] The future will undoubtedly bring increasingly significant challenges to our understanding of the nature of medicine. In response, Christian doctors may choose to form a sub-culture within medicine as distinctive as that of their Hippocratic forebears. Such a move may be critical since medicine as we have known it will cease to exist if medical techniques are divorced from moral commitment.

3. How do I choose a physician whom I can trust?

This question is difficult to address and must be examined from a number of perspectives. We believe that most physicians can be trusted. It's unfortunate, however, that a small minority of physicians are unethical and/or uncaring. Some patients have had bad experiences with certain doctors, which can negatively influence those patients' perceptions of the whole healthcare profession. It's important, though, to recognize that physicians must complete many years of education that often cost them tens of thousands of dollars, endure incredibly long hours during residency, and deal with enormous stress in their day-to-day practices. Most physicians were, therefore, motivated to enter the field of medicine because they truly wanted to help people, and they continue to practice because of this desire. Nevertheless, patients should take all possible steps to ensure that they choose physicians who are trustworthy.

The trust you need to have in your physician will vary with your reasons for visiting him or her. If, for example, you have a condition that you suspect might require surgery, your main selection criteria will likely be a physician's ability to diagnose your condition correctly and to perform or make available surgical procedures as appropriate. Your choice of physician may be limited, though, by whoever is covered by your insurance, or you may have to rely on the recommendations of your primary care physician (your family doctor).

Such reliance underscores the importance of trusting your primary care physician and emphasizes the necessity of choosing a good one. Before selecting a primary care doctor, you might begin by asking family members and friends for their recommendations. If this is not possible, it would be wise to speak with current patients of prospective physicians.

Before selecting a physician, it's helpful to make appointments to see a few. Many physicians are open to scheduling appointments for the sole purpose of meeting potential new patients. A physician who's willing to take the time to do this will also likely take the time to discuss important questions you may have later on about your health or treatment options. Before visiting a prospective physician, prepare some questions to bring with you. These questions will vary depending upon your stage of life. You may, for instance, want to know about your doctor's views on contraception or end-of-life care if these issues are likely to arise in the near future.

As with most relationships, it is only by getting to know your doctor that you'll learn whether or not you can trust him or her. Take notice of how your physician treats you and responds to you. Does he or she listen to you, explain things to you, and assist you in reaching decisions with which you're comfortable? Developing trust requires that both parties in a relationship exhibit certain attitudes and

17

behaviors. Thus, patients should be open with their physicians about the concerns they have and be honest about the things they are doing in their lives, especially those behaviors that are not the most healthy. Physicians should likewise reflect honesty and openness in interacting with their patients.

It is an unfortunate possibility, however, that at some point your trust in your physician may diminish. If you can discuss the problematic issues immediately, you may be able to move your relationship back onto better footing. If, however, you cannot, you may need to find another physician in whom you can have more trust. Given the importance and delicacy of many of the matters that may arise between a patient and a physician, trust is worth building and maintaining, even if this requires beginning again with a new physician. We must always remember that our doctors are human and that they are challenged by many different commitments. This makes it all the more important, though, that patients place a high priority on choosing doctors whom they are able to trust.

4. How important is it for a Christian patient to see a Christian doctor?

People differ widely in their beliefs concerning the role of faith and religion in healthcare. Some individuals view the human body as essentially a machine that must be repaired from time to time. Machines can be fixed, of course, without any consideration of spiritual matters. In this mechanistic view, healing is equated solely with the correction of biological dysfunction, as is the case in veterinary medicine. Those who hold this view will likely pay little or no attention to the emotional and spiritual dimensions of healing. On the other hand, some people place great emphasis on the non-physical aspects of health and disease.

In recent years, many societies have become increasingly comprised of people with diverse worldviews. In Western culture, the influence of the Christian worldview has decreased. Accordingly, Christians cannot assume that their doctors will share their faith. Sharing similar bonds of faith would perhaps be less important if the practice of medicine were primarily an enterprise requiring only technical knowledge and skill in using medical instruments. If such were the case, one knowledgeable physician would, in essence, be like any other. The practice of medicine, though, extends far beyond the level of technical knowledge and skill.

Many of the most difficult issues in medicine are moral in that the questions involve wrestling with what is right and wrong (e.g., in the realm of abortion and reproductive technology, genetic intervention, and end-of-life decision-making); therefore, the decision-making process will likely be smoother if both the doctor and patient share the same religious beliefs. In such cases, issues of concern can be discussed directly in the light of Christian faith and decisions made only after prayerful consideration. Christian patients should always be discerning when physicians offer spiritual advice, especially if they recommend alternative therapies of a spiritual origin. Christians are called to test all spirits to see if they are from God (1 John 4:1–3), and that includes those involved in treatments offered in the name of healing (see the *Alternative Medicine* booklet in this series).

Since Christian physicians should be best suited to address the spiritual aspect of a patient's life, it may seem logical to assume that Christian patients should select Christian doctors whenever possible. But should Christians always seek such an arrangement, or are there times when having a Christian doctor is not of primary importance? In some medical situations, ethical issues loom large, while in others a doctor's personal beliefs make little difference. Some examples of the latter would include the receipt of anesthesia, certain surgeries, and much of preventive medicine (although many lifestyle issues affecting health do involve ethics). Other situations—emergency situations, geographical constraints, particular healthcare plans—may limit a patient's choice of physicians. In situations like these, the availability of a competent physician may be more important than whether or not the doctor is a Christian.

Generally speaking, however, there are many advantages to having a Christian doctor. Christian physicians are called to practice medicine in a specific way. They should exhibit particular characteristics and follow certain principles that are based on their relationship with Christ and on the recognition that human life is sacred because it is created in the very image of God. To provide effective care to patients, Christian physicians are to view Jesus, who spent a great deal of time healing the sick, as their guide. When He sent His disciples out to proclaim the kingdom in Matthew 10:5–10, healing was a key sign of the reality of the coming kingdom. For these reasons, Christian doctors have a responsibility through prayer and the study of Scripture to seek to discern the applications of their beliefs to their clinical practice.

Although non-Christian physicians are often very fine doctors, your physician may be more likely to share your values and ethics if he or she is also a Christian. To find a good Christian physician, you might ask people at your church for suggestions or check your local Christian business directory. Another option is the Christian Medical & Dental Associations (CMDA), which publishes on their Web site the names, phone numbers, and specialties of CMDA members who have chosen to be listed. The site may be accessed at http://www.cmdahome.org, and the physicians list can be searched by state by clicking on the "search" icon.

Provided that professional competence is not compromised, a covenant between a Christian patient and Christian doctor would likely be the ideal scenario.

5. What is a parish nurse, and why do some churches have one?

In general, parish nurses are registered nurses who practice *holistic* healthcare within a particular congregation. The term *holistic* conveys the recognition that spiritual, psychological, relational, and physical aspects of a patient's life are important to his or her health and healing. Parish nurses particularly stress the importance of spirituality and faith for health. A parish nurse performs a variety of roles depending upon the nature and philosophy of the particular nurse, as well as upon the organization that oversees his or her practice. Parish nurses are generally not involved in providing traditional nursing care to very ill members of the community. Rather, parish nurses typically offer programs in health education, conduct health screenings, refer people to traditional healthcare professionals, and help people to integrate their faith with issues of healthcare. Parish nurses may volunteer their time, or they may be employed by a church or healthcare organization.

The American Nurses Association designated parish nursing as a specialty practice in 1997. About two thousand parish nurses are certified in the U.S. and practice within Roman Catholic, Protestant, and Jewish congregations. Although interest in parish nursing is a relatively new phenomenon in the United States, it represents a return to the original roots of nursing as it developed within religious communities. Parish nursing fulfills the desire of many

21

nurses to help meet the healthcare needs of their faith community. For them, it is a way to integrate their professional training with their commitment to minister to others.

Christians, too, should affirm the importance of faith for health. All illness is ultimately the result of the Fall, which brought about spiritual alienation between all of humanity and God. Jesus Christ came to bring healing to human beings, which included the physical healing evidenced in His many miracles. Jesus' primary focus, however, was on *spiritual* healing, which comes through renewed spiritual life. "I have come that they may have life, and have it to the full" (John 10:10). Contrary to much of popular belief in our culture, Jesus did not teach that people can achieve spiritual health through whatever paths they choose. He taught, rather, that spiritual health comes only through a relationship with Him and through obedience to God (John 15:14).

This exclusivity leads to a major concern some people have with parish nursing. As stated earlier, parish nursing is based on a *holistic* philosophy of health and healing. The term "holistic" can, however, mean different things to different people. Holistic health has been interpreted by some to include any form of spirituality—whether Christian, Hindu, New Age, or whatever. The worldviews of some parish nurses may lead them to recommend spiritual practices or complementary and alternative therapies that are intimately tied into non-Christian religious beliefs. (These issues are discussed in more detail in the *Alternative Medicine* booklet in this series.) Therefore, before engaging the services of a parish nurse, Christian individuals and churches should carefully explore a nurse's particular view of spirituality and exactly what he or she means by "holistic health."

Parish nurses who practice within a biblical worldview may provide very valuable resources to the community. Their professional training enables them to educate people about healthcare and to recognize when people have early symptoms of disease and would likely benefit from visiting their doctors sooner rather than later. In addition, people may be more open with a parish nurse than with other healthcare professionals about concerns they have regarding their spiritual growth and how it may be impacting their health or personal relationships. Parish nurses can also discuss with their patients the value of Bible reading and meditation, prayer, fellowship with other Christians, and service as related to personal well-being.

In summary, parish nursing brings nurses back to the spiritual roots of their profession and provides nurses with practical ways to put their faith into action. As such, parish nurses can serve as excellent examples to others in the Church, encouraging them to examine how their own professional training and talents may be put to good use within their congregations.

CAREGIVER-PATIENT COMMUNICATION

---

6. How important is it for physicians to tell their patients the truth?

Telling patients the truth is essential if physicians are to develop trusting physician/patient relationships. Patients often feel very vulnerable when they visit their doctors regarding illnesses from which they are suffering or pain that they are experiencing. Some patients are willing to accept whatever course of action their physicians suggest, especially if they have been highly recommended and/or are widely recognized for their expertise within a particular area of medicine. Some patients may also be too intimidated to ask questions if they view their physicians as authority figures or experts. Because of patients' inherent vulnerability and their need to trust, physicians are ethically obligated to seek always to act in their patients' best interests. This obligation raises the question of how the best interests of patients may be determined and whether such interests include being told the truth.

In the past, many physicians and patients readily accepted the notion of *paternalism:* the idea that the doctor knows best (see question 7). Even today, some patients prefer that their doctors make important and difficult medical decisions for them. Most people, however, have been influenced by the contemporary emphasis on *individual autonomy,* which regards the patient as the primary (and often sole) decision-maker regarding healthcare decisions. As a result, physicians are increasingly viewed as their patients' advocates, helping patients decide what is in their own best interests.

Due in part to this shift in medical decision-making, the notion of *informed consent* (see question 7) has become an important ethical value in medicine. In order for patients to make wise healthcare decisions, they must be given accurate information. Herein lies the connection to truth-telling. To ensure that a patient is able to give informed consent for a treatment or procedure, the physician must be truthful about the patient's diagnosis, the benefits and risks of available interventions, and any other relevant matters. Truthfulness is thus foundational to the ethical practice of medicine today.

Some people wonder, however, if physicians may ethically refrain from telling the truth. One such situation might be when a doctor fears that telling the truth may actually be harmful to the patient. A physician may fear, for example, that telling an elderly patient she has cancer might diminish her will to live. Such an outcome might be especially likely to arise if nothing can be done for the patient medically. Upon learning her diagnosis, the patient might become severely depressed and die sooner than she otherwise would. In a case like this, would the doctor be justified in not telling the patient that she has cancer? If the patient directly asked for her diagnosis, should the doctor lie about it? These questions are posed with the assumption that the doctor is motivated completely out of concern for his patient's well-being.

The problem with lying to patients, or withholding the truth from them, is that it reflects a very limited view of patients' well-being. If a patient has a relatively short length of time to live, he or she may indeed become depressed but may also seize the opportunity to address unresolved emotional, relational, and spiritual issues. Moreover, research has indicated that seriously ill patients often have a good idea about the nature of their condition prior to receiving a diagnosis. If doctors are not forthright with the truth, patients may become even more depressed, worrying that their conditions are worse than they'd feared.

Christian physicians should also be concerned about the image they project to patients and their families, and whether it accurately reflects the character of God. Throughout Scripture, God places a strong emphasis on truth. God is Himself called a "God of truth" (Ps. 31:5), and the psalmist declared that God desires us to have truth in our "inner parts" (Ps. 51:6). Jesus also told us that the "truth will set [us] free" (John 8:32). Furthermore, God has not held back in revealing His diagnosis of our spiritual condition, which is far more dire than any physical diagnosis could ever be. It's not surprising, then, that failure to tell the truth usually has negative consequences. Patients and family members who discover that their physicians withheld information from them, or lied to them, may be significantly hurt and find it difficult to trust their doctors in the future. Although patients may, indeed, react negatively to the truth, it is almost always in their best interests to hear it.

While disclosing the truth to patients is usually best, physicians will occasionally encounter a situation where they know a patient well enough to determine with confidence that telling him or her the truth would be unwise because significant harm to the patient or others would likely result. The truth should only be withheld, however, after much prayer and deliberation and following consultation with other professionals. Informing other family members about a patient's condition without informing the patient should also only be done with great hesitation, and only under the exceptional circumstances when a breach of patient confidentiality is justified (see questions 11 and 13). Telling the truth is so important to the formation of trusting relationships that it should be withheld or distorted only under the most severe conditions.

Whether it is the right or wrong course of action, physicians who withhold the truth are usually well-intentioned. Sometimes, though, a physician will withhold—or even distort—the truth for reasons that are entirely self-serving. If, for example, a physician knows that a patient is worried about undergoing a procedure that other doctors have presented as his only option, the physician may challenge the necessity of the procedure and recommend a much less painful or invasive intervention—even if she knows full well that the feared procedure will ultimately be necessary. By doing so, the physician may stand to benefit financially if the patient selects her as his healthcare professional based upon her offering him a more attractive option than have other doctors. Once he's chosen this physician, he will likely remain with her when she informs him that the more attractive intervention has failed to alleviate the problem and that the dreaded procedure is, after all, necessary. Although we may never encounter a physician who withholds or distorts the truth in an attempt to achieve personal gain, we should guard against this possibility by seeking multiple opinions before making major healthcare decisions—regardless of a physician's reputation or skill.

Finally, a physician's commitment to telling the truth should always be coupled with concern for how the truth is presented. Paul urges us to "speak the truth in love" (see Eph. 4:15). Physicians should carefully and sensitively time their presentation of the truth and should do their utmost to break difficult news with gentleness and empathy. Since a doctor will be required to move on to other patients at some point following the delivery of a troubling diagnosis, he or she should arrange ahead of time to have others (such as chaplains or social workers) ready to remain with the patient, providing comfort and counsel once the doctor has departed.

7. What is "informed consent"?

Informed consent, simply described, is permission given by patients or their surrogates to accept a medical intervention following physician disclosure of the nature of the intervention, its potential benefits and risks, and the available alternatives and their potential benefits and risks. Since treatment options almost always carry both potential benefits and risks and patients are given the right to make decisions about their healthcare, it is important for patients to be able to make informed choices. Before identifying the conditions that must be met in order for a patient's consent to be truly informed—and discussing the implications of such consent—it will be helpful to review how this concept came to be accepted as a fundamental principle in bioethics.

In the past, people were often given scanty information about their medical conditions, and physicians, as the experts, typically decided what was in the patients' best interests. Since the physician (then usually a male) made decisions for his patients much like a father would for his children, this mode of decision-making came to be known as *paternalism.*

With the 1960s came an increased emphasis on patients' rights. This development coincided with technological advances such as kidney dialysis machines and mechanical respirators, which could prolong life indefinitely yet, in some cases, without hope for improvement. Many people believed that it wasn't right to impose such interventions on patients against their wills. In a relatively few years, a social and ethical consensus developed that patients should have ultimate control over whether to accept medical treatments offered by their doctors. The physician's responsibility thus shifted from making decisions for patients to providing sufficient information about the nature of their diseases, the intended benefits and risks of the recommended treatment, and the benefits and risks of alternative treatments. Patients could then make their own informed healthcare decisions.

It soon became clear that multiple conditions had to be met for a patient's decision to be truly informed and morally valid. The following four criteria need to be considered when determining whether informed consent has been given:

1. *Competence or Capacity.* Incompetent or mentally compromised patients may not be able to make rational decisions about what is in their best interests. Before honoring a patient's expressed wishes, a doctor must determine (to the best of his or her ability) that the patient is capable of making sound decisions. In evaluating a patient's mental capacity ("competence" is the legal term for this) the physician should ask questions like:

   - Is the patient able to understand conversations?
   - Does the patient have the ability to understand the disease process and to rationally weigh the different treatment options?
   - Can the patient place his or her treatment choices in the context of his or her value system?

   Sometimes the determination of mental competence is straightforward, and sometimes it's so difficult that a psychiatric consultation is needed. It may also be necessary to ask if any co-existing conditions (mental illness, drug side-effects, etc.) are present that could be affecting rational cognitive function.

2. *Freedom of Choice.* To have moral standing, a choice must be free. Coercion unduly influences and can invalidate a patient's decision. Physicians must be aware of this danger both in their own conversations with patients and with regard to patients' discussions with other healthcare professionals and families and friends. Physicians must recognize that there is a fine line between advising and encouraging ill persons and pressuring them.

3. *Information.* This is obviously a critical ingredient in informed consent. Information provided to a patient

must include the nature of his or her condition, the purpose of the proposed treatment or procedure, and a discussion of the risks and potential benefits associated with this intervention. A discussion of other possible therapies, along with their associated potential benefits and risks, must also take place. The doctor has an ethical obligation to discuss such alternatives with the patient, regardless of whether the physician feels that they are cost-effective or whether the interventions in question are covered by the patient's healthcare plan. The risks and potential benefits of not receiving any treatment at all should also be discussed.

4. *Understanding.* This criterion is often neglected; yet without an adequate understanding on the patient's part, meeting the first three criteria will prove to be meaningless. Sometimes a competent patient will seem to listen to her doctor carefully, but due to other concerns will fail to understand some of the vital implications of the information being provided. At the very least, patients must be given the opportunity to ask relevant questions. Discussing various options with patients and asking them to put into their own words what they have been told can confirm how well they understand what has been communicated.

Physicians indeed have a duty to ensure that all four requirements of informed consent are satisfied, followed by patient authorization (usually via the patient's signature). In affirming this duty, it should be noted that the extent of information to be provided is not precisely clear. For example, some drugs may have dozens of potential side-effects that only very rarely occur. Is a doctor required to communicate to patients each and every one even if the actual occurrence is highly unlikely? The answer to this question is no; however, physicians lack generally agreed upon guidelines regarding risk disclosure other than that any serious or reasonably likely risk should be discussed.

In closing, two exceptions to informed consent are noted:

1. In emergency situations in which a patient is incapable of providing informed consent and no one else is available to speak for him or her, the doctor must make decisions about treatment. If harm from a failure to treat is imminent and outweighs the likelihood and degree of harm from the proposed intervention, then the physician should proceed with the treatment.
2. Situations occasionally arise in which physicians feel that divulging certain information would be harmful to their patients and/or would complicate the treatment. These are difficult scenarios because of the importance of truth-telling for developing trust between physicians and patients (see question 6 for further elaboration). If a doctor decides not to obtain a patient's fully informed consent, he or she should have sound medical grounds for concluding that a discussion of the disease process and treatment options poses a serious risk to the patient's well-being. In such situations, physicians should obtain a second opinion and carefully document the reasoning behind their decisions since, should a dispute later ensue, they would likely bear the burden of proof that withholding information was necessary.

In summary, patients' preferences with regard to medical treatment are morally significant and should be respected. Informed consent serves to equip patients to make decisions about their healthcare and to ensure that they've been provided with relevant information regarding particular medical interventions.

8. Should physicians ever order treatment that they know is against their patients' wishes?

This question should be approached by expanding the previous discussion of *informed consent* (see answer to question 7). If a patient has refused to consent to a medical intervention and the criteria of "competence/capacity," "freedom of choice," "information," and "understanding" have been satisfied, then it is unethical to administer treatment against the patient's wishes. Many situations occur, however, in which it is not clear whether a patient's refusal of treatment is rational and informed.

When patients are incompetent, their physicians may believe that they are ethically required to administer treatment. For example, if a psychotic paranoid patient believes that all medicine is a form of deadly poison and therefore refuses treatment, a physician may feel that it is his duty to provide treatment anyway due to the patient's incompetence to make medical decisions. Most states, though, have laws addressing such situations that often require physicians to obtain court orders to overrule such treatment refusals. Such is the seriousness given to patients' rights to make their own decisions.

Other cases involving determination of a patient's competence are even more challenging. For example, in situations in which a chronically ill patient becomes depressed and requests that all therapy cease, decisions about whether to honor such a request may be extremely difficult. Is a depressed patient competent to refuse life-saving therapy in the same way that a rational, non-depressed patient is? Most physicians would say no. In situations like this, there is a fine line between rightly honoring a patient's expressed wishes and allowing a depressed patient in a confused mental state to stop life-sustaining treatments when he or she should be prevented from doing so. In such cases, it is sometimes necessary to evaluate a patient's competence over a period of time, rather than immediately agreeing to his or her stated desires.

It is also important to recognize that a patient's refusal to begin therapy or a request to stop ongoing therapy may result from pressure or coercion from others. If the patient's family members, hospital administrators, or third party payers decide that the patient's life is not worth living, is an imposition on the family, or is too costly for the medical system, then the patient may feel prompted to refuse therapy. In situations like these, the physician has a moral obligation to protect the patient, which may require closely ascertaining the motives behind his or her requests. If refusal of therapy does actually arise from external pressure, the requirements for informed medical decision-making (which include "free choice") have not been met and the doctor has a moral obligation to address the attempted coercion. An ethics consultation/committee may be helpful for carrying out such a process (see questions 15–17).

Physicians must make sure their patients have met the four criteria for informed consent before making decisions concerning treatment. In the event that all criteria have been satisfied, physicians are ultimately required to honor patients' expressed desires and should commit their patients to God, who will wisely judge all hearts. To do otherwise would be to deny the patients' decision-making responsibilities as moral agents created in the image of God.

9. Is it appropriate for doctors and other healthcare professionals to talk with their patients about spiritual issues?

One of the major developments within medicine at the end of the twentieth century was the renewed interest in spirituality and the impact it has on health. Books like David and Susan Larson's *The Forgotten Factor in Physical and Mental Health: What Does the Research Show?* and Dale Matthews' *The Faith Factor* consider more than two hundred studies demonstrating that patients who have religious or spiritual beliefs often enjoy better health and longer life and demonstrate an enhanced ability to cope with illness.[3] In addition, the *Handbook of Religion and Health* by Harold G. Koenig, Michael McCullough, and David Larson summarizes in a comprehensive fashion the research and literature on the relationship between religion and health.[4]

Prompted in part by these scientific findings, professional medical journals began to debate whether physicians should prescribe prayer and religious involvement as a means of improving their patients' health. The broader question here is whether doctors should discuss spiritual issues with their patients in addition to addressing medical concerns. Surveys consistently reveal that a majority of patients want their physicians to raise spiritual matters with them. In one study, two-thirds of the patients surveyed believed that physician/patient relationships would improve if physicians asked patients about their religious and spiritual beliefs.[5] This same study found that half of those who considered themselves to be non-religious would, nevertheless, like their physicians to discuss spiritual issues with them in certain situations. Studies show, however, that in practice, physicians rarely address matters of faith with their patients.

Patients—especially those who are seriously ill or dying—often have questions about why they are suffering, questions that extend beyond the medical reasons for their afflictions. Instead of merely receiving a medical prognosis, they may desire counsel as to how they can cope with resulting limitations or disabilities. They may also want to know what will happen once their lives are over.

Although patients often desire religious and spiritual answers to their questions, doctors often prefer to focus on providing information that is strictly medical in nature. Many physicians feel that they are not adequately trained to address spiritual concerns. Although medicine and religion were intimately connected throughout much of human history, spiritual issues were left largely to religion as medicine became more science-based and specialized. At the same time, the Church moved away from its role in healthcare and focused more on meeting people's spiritual needs. At the beginning of the twenty-first century, there is a growing interest in bringing matters of faith and medicine together again.

It is still true, however, that doctors, nurses, and other healthcare professionals are usually better prepared to address medical, rather than spiritual, issues. Often such persons may have no answers to spiritual questions, even for themselves. So, if healthcare professionals were to address spiritual needs, they might not do so as well as would "spiritual specialists." Thus, hospitals and nursing homes employ chaplains; and pastors, rabbis, and priests commit themselves to visiting the sick. It is an unfortunate fact, however, that many chaplains are not comfortable with what they perceive as "traditional religion" and instead promote a more generalized form of spirituality, which they recommend that patients adapt to suit their individual needs.

Some people fear that if doctors and nurses were to address spiritual issues, the patient-professional relationship would be negatively impacted. Physicians, especially, have a significant level of power over their patients, whether or not this is acknowledged. Physicians are authority figures, and patients often feel very vulnerable when they are sick, confused, or afraid. Consequently, some patients may feel compelled to accept the spiritual beliefs or practices of their physicians due to a perceived inappropriateness of challenging someone of such stature, or out of fear that they may not be treated as well if they disagree with those who are providing their care. Some people therefore believe that physicians should limit their spiritual discussions with patients to mere acknowledgment of the patients' concerns.

Such an approach fails to recognize, however, the importance of providing spiritual answers to people's spiritual questions. Just as healthcare professionals seek to provide the best healthcare possible, they should be willing to point their patients to the best spiritual care possible, which is that found in Jesus Christ. When Christian caregivers are asked by their patients about spiritual matters, they shouldn't avoid providing them with specific input. They can respond by sharing personally or by connecting them with other people and/or ministries who have the knowledge and time to answer their questions. Patients who ask for spiritual direction should be presented with the truth of biblical Christianity, although precisely what is presented should be determined by the specific context. While not holding back such truth, Christian healthcare professionals should, indeed, be sensitive to any authority issues that their patients may have and must take steps to ensure that patients do not feel coerced into accepting their caregivers' beliefs. At the same time, caregivers should make it clear that their beliefs are not just ones that "work for them," but that they are God's truths and are true for everyone. Christian healthcare professionals should direct patients to passages in the Bible where they can read such truths for themselves and should also encourage patients to pray and seek a personal relationship with Christ.

Christian caregivers must also accept that healthcare professionals of different faiths likewise have the freedom to share their religious beliefs with their patients. Christian caregivers should encourage dialogue between people of different faiths, while not giving in to the idea that all religions are equally true. Such a notion reflects a lack of knowledge about the significant differences between the major world religions; therefore, to assert such differences does *not* translate into a lack of tolerance. To be truly tolerant, rather, we must maintain that there are differences between people's religious beliefs and then show respect for those people who do not share our convictions. If, however, we refuse to address the different viewpoints concerning how people receive salvation, then we may leave some patients to suffer the consequences of not accepting Jesus Christ as their Savior.

10. Is it okay to ask a doctor who is not a Christian to pray with me?

When a person is ill or injured, it is entirely appropriate to pray for healing. In fact, James 5 instructs Christians to pray for one another when illness arises and to call the elders to anoint and pray for those who are ill. While this passage clearly instructs Christians to pray for healing, should a Christian patient ask a non-Christian doctor (or other healthcare professional) to pray with him or her? Would such a doctor's prayers be effective? Might the doctor pray to a god other than the patient's God?

The question concerning the efficacy of a non-Christian doctor's prayer can be resolved theologically by reflecting on the fact that God does listen to the prayers of those who are not Christians. Prior to becoming Christians, many people have prayed for and received God's help and insight. Consider also that all Christians had to pray—as non-Christians—in order to become Christians, and God certainly answered those prayers. Prayer is simply communication with God, and, as such, God wants those who are Christians and those who are not Christians to pray to Him.

Christian patients should realize that praying with a doctor who might not share their faith could be an important witness. A doctor will likely expect a patient's prayer to include requests for her own health and comfort. The doctor may therefore be surprised if the prayer also expresses concern for him and others on the healthcare team, for the difficult decisions that everyone must make, and for the well-being of everyone involved in caring for the patient. Prayers of gratitude for the people caring for the patient and for the sacrifices they make on her behalf might likely touch the doctor's heart and spirit. Prayers of confidence in God's love and the hope of eternity within the patient may communicate far more to a busy doctor than a gospel tract ever would. Praying with a doctor who is not a Christian would thus seem to be entirely appropriate and should even be encouraged.

Christian patients should be careful, however, to convey what they mean when raising the issue of prayer with a doctor who is not a Christian. The patient should make it clear that he or she is inviting the doctor to be present with the patient as that person prays to *his or her* God. It should *not* be seen as a general invitation for everyone present to pray to whatever gods they believe in. The first Commandment is to put no other gods before God (Exod. 20:3). Paul also warned the Corinthians not to participate in any form of idol worship (1 Cor. 10:20–22). Furthermore, contacting spirits other than God is completely forbidden (Deut. 18:10–14) and is profoundly dangerous (1 Peter 5:8). Yet Christians must also remember that their God is greater than all other gods (1 John 4:4) and should not fear His rejection, as nothing can come between them and His love (Rom. 8:38–39).

Physicians should also be given the freedom to refuse a patient's invitation to be present during prayer. A patient could issue such an invitation in the following manner: "I am a Christian and would like to pray before we proceed. I would love to have you stay and join me, but I don't know your religious beliefs and don't want to push you into something that would make you uncomfortable. Would you like to stay with me while I pray?" This would give the doctor the freedom to leave, to stay in silence, or to join in the prayer, and would also resolve concerns a patient might have about the appropriateness of initiating prayer in the presence of people who do not (or might not) know God. It might also be the beginning of an opportunity for a Christian patient to share the hope that is within her (1 Peter 3:15).

At the end of the twentieth century, medicine began to rediscover the importance of spirituality to health. As a consequence, many non-believing doctors now have a greater appreciation for the importance of respecting and supporting their patients' religious beliefs. Initiating prayer with a doctor today will often be received more positively than it would have been just a couple of decades ago (see question 9). Still, Christian patients are sometimes reluctant to mention prayer for fear that doctors might react negatively or dismiss prayer as unimportant and ineffective. Today's physicians, though, are more likely to recognize the value some patients place on prayer, regardless of what the doctors' own religious beliefs might be. Therefore, Christians should make the most of the current openness to matters of spirituality among healthcare professionals. They should confidently and openly invite doctors to join them in spiritual discussions and prayer, while doing their best to ensure that any prayer that occurs is directed only to the one true God.

11. Is my physician obligated to keep information about my health and medical history confidential?

The tenets of both the American Medical Association (AMA) and the Hippocratic Oath, considered binding by many physicians, require doctors to keep private patient information confidential. Physicians' legal obligations regarding confidentiality are ultimately rooted in the U.S. Constitution, as well as in federal and state law. Most courts allow legal action to be taken against doctors who divulge confidential medical information without proper authorization from the patient.

In spite of these protections, changes in the way medicine is practiced and patient data is stored have led to situations where patient confidentiality has been unintentionally compromised. Today, medicine is practiced in an integrated healthcare system through which multiple healthcare professionals and medical students have access to patients' medical information. Moreover, this information is stored in data banks and clinical registries. The purpose of compiling and storing this information is generally valid, as systematic reviews of these records may result in better, more efficient patient care. Managed care organizations, for example, insist upon reviewing patients' medical records to determine if particular treatments are warranted. National organizations that accredit hospitals and physician specialty groups also insist on studying medical records as a means of determining the appropriateness and completeness of medical record-keeping and physicians' note-taking. In addition, the government is currently reviewing private medical records as a means of obtaining information that will allow more effective allocation of funds for patient care and research. Further, more law enforcement agencies are also accessing patient records in order to detect medical fraud (although they must obtain legal authorization, such as a warrant, subpoena, or summons, before doing so). While all of these purposes may be well-intentioned, patient confidentiality is nevertheless, compromised. Consequently, the AMA, as well as others, have serious concerns about breaches of patient confidentiality.

In theory, your medical records may only be released to others after you have provided written authorization for such disclosure. You must give permission in order for your records to be released to your attorney, insurance company, employer, or even to a family member. Such a policy is based upon respect for patient privacy, the desire to protect patients from harm or discrimination, and the critical need to maintain a bond of trust between patients and their doctors. If physicians cannot be trusted by their patients to keep details about their health and/or medical conditions private, a patient may be unwilling to share information that is essential in order for the physician to deliver the best possible care to that patient.

Situations do exist, however, in which a patient's consent to share information is implied, such as when that patient is hospitalized or is transferred from one institution to another. In these circumstances, sharing of confidential patient information may be necessary to ensure continuation of that patient's care; therefore, consent may be presumed. Other circumstances also exist in which the protection of confidentiality must give way to competing interests. While the complete list varies from state to state, physicians may be legally mandated to report such things as weapon-related injuries, infectious diseases, and suspected child abuse. In addition, when dealing with emotionally distraught patients who are threatening to seriously harm themselves or others, therapists may be required to disclose such threats to appropriate law enforcement officers and the intended victims.[6] In such cases, the legislatures and the court system have determined that the need to protect innocent lives overrides concerns about patient confidentiality. The following set of guidelines is designed to help a physician or therapist recognize a situation in which it's necessary to breach patient or client confidentiality and share private medical or personal information with others:

1. The likelihood is significant that harm will come to someone unless the information is divulged.
2. Releasing the information seems likely to prevent the harm.
3. The decision to divulge the information is made only after attempts to persuade the patient to disclose the information himself or herself have failed.
4. It would seem reasonable to breach the confidentiality of *any* patient in the given situation.

Aside from these exceptional circumstances, the recent trend toward increased disclosure of identifiable patient information apart from patient consent is of growing concern to those who might be affected. The greatest danger is that this information will become available to organizations that could be tempted to use it for discriminatory purposes. For example, employers could make hiring decisions based on access to an individual's private medical record, or banks could turn down requests for loans based upon a person's medical history.

Since April 14, 2003, extensive new guidelines known as HIPAA (Health Insurance Portability and Accountability Act) have been in place to protect the privacy of patients' medical records (see http://aspe.hhs.gov/admnsimp). Further discussion regarding the intent of these regulations can be found at www.healthprivacy.org.

12. What is a medical record, and do I have access to mine?

Medical records contain documentations of medical treatment or formal advice that a patient has received from a physician, nurse, or other healthcare professional. Your medical records may include your medical history, family medical history, and general information about your lifestyle that you've provided in discussions with your healthcare professionals. Your medical records may also contain x-ray results, laboratory test results, and details concerning any operations or procedures that you have undergone. If you have ever been hospitalized, the admission record will also contain additional notes supplied by your physician, nurses, and other healthcare professionals.

There are many valid reasons why you should have access to your medical records. These include the need to feel confident that your physician is not keeping information from you that you may wish to see. By willingly showing you the contents of your medical records, your physician will further build a basis of trust and openness. It is also important for healthcare professionals to understand that, while a patient's medical records may belong to her, the data in the records should, nevertheless, be made available to the patient on request.

On April 14, 2003, the Health Insurance Portability and Accountability Act (HIPAA) became fully effective in the United States. One of the sections of this Act establishes a new federal legal right for patients to see and obtain a copy of their medical records. In general, the physician, hospital, or other entity responsible for maintaining a patient's medical records has thirty days to honor his request to inspect or obtain a copy of his records. In certain circumstances, this thirty-day deadline may be extended to sixty days provided that the patient is given a written explanation for the further delay. There are, however, several grounds for denying access to medical records, and an appeals process may also be employed in such instances. (For more information, see www.healthprivacy.org/usr_doc/SummaryReg2002.pdf.)

If you should desire a copy of your medical records, inform your doctor's office or hospital. Because medical records do belong to such settings, the facility may charge you a fee for locating and copying your records. In most states, it's relatively easy for patients to obtain their medical records or at least the pertinent portions. Be aware, though, that a variety of state laws govern the release of medical records and some states have more rigorous standards for making medical records available. In such cases, the stricter state laws take precedence over the federal standard. Most states require patients to sign a release form that frees from responsibility the one providing the medical records should a breach of confidentiality occur because the patient has been provided with a copy of her records.

If you have any difficulty in obtaining your medical records, call your state's department of health for specific governing regulations. As an alternative, you might wish to access www.healthprivacy.org on the Internet. This site contains a substantive report documenting the appropriate regulations in each of the fifty states.

13. If my adolescent goes to the doctor, can I as a parent find out what kind of information was shared and what kind of care was provided?

Adolescence is a time of transition from childhood to adulthood. People may be referred to as adolescents from the time they are twelve years old until their eighteenth birthday (or until they reach "legal age").

Confidential care for adolescent patients means that the physician will not reveal any information to anyone (including the patient's parents) without the adolescent's consent. This is particularly important since adolescents are often more willing to discuss sensitive issues (such as sexual behavior and/or sexually transmitted diseases, substance abuse, and psychological problems) with their physician when they have the assurance of confidentiality. If an adolescent is legally emancipated or determined by a court to be sufficiently mature, confidentiality regarding an abortion procedure may be protected even if doing so requires bypassing state parental consent or notice provisions.

In providing healthcare, physicians must strive to balance the growing independence of their adolescent patients with the reality that they are still dependent upon their parents in many ways and that it is the parents' responsibility to ensure that their adolescents receive appropriate care. Although confidentiality may understandably be an important concern for adolescents, parental involvement in an adolescent's healthcare is almost always beneficial and should therefore be encouraged. Good communication among all involved parties is vital. Many physicians will therefore initiate discussions about confidentiality with adolescent patients and their parents, outlining what types of information they will not disclose to parents as well as situations in which confidentiality may be broken due to the potential risk to the adolescent and/or others. Physicians should also inform their adolescent patients that medical billing issues often impact confidentiality. In the case of diagnosis and treatment of sexually transmitted diseases, for example, it should be made clear that laboratory and medical bills would be sent directly to the parents of the adolescent unless he or she makes arrangements to self-pay for such services.

In actual practice, one or both parents are most often present at younger adolescents' medical appointments. It is common for physicians to select a certain age (for example, thirteen) and communicate prior to that time that once a patient reaches this age, his or her parents may continue to be present during the information-gathering portion of an office visit but not during the examination itself. Following their child's examination, parents will typically be invited back into the exam room to discuss any diagnosis, prognosis, and recommended treatment. Such an approach allows the physician to build a relationship with the adolescent that is independent of the parental relationship, thereby facilitating the young person's transition to fully independent decision-making. At the same time, this approach respects and promotes the importance of the parent-adolescent relationship.

An American Medical Association (AMA) bulletin reports that, under the new HIPAA provisions (see questions 11 and 12), if a parent is not the legal representative of a minor and the state or other law is silent or unclear [regarding confidentiality], discretion to provide or deny a parent access to the minor's protected health information may rest with the physician/provider.[7] Some state laws do protect confidentiality explicitly with respect to contraception, treatment for pregnancy, abortion, testing for STDs and HIV, mental health treatment, and/or eating disorders.

Military regulations provide confidentiality for patients thirteen and over for mental health and substance abuse issues; and patients fourteen and over may receive confidential care for contraception, possible pregnancy, and sexually transmitted diseases.

Similarly, many professional organizations recommend protecting adolescent confidentiality in order to provide better care, particularly with regard to psychiatric care, substance abuse, sexual activity, and dysfunctional family environments. From a legal standpoint, however, the bottom line is that parents *can* in most cases find out what transpired during their adolescents' doctors' appointments. This fact could have the unfortunate consequence of jeopardizing the medical care of adolescents if they withhold important medical information out of fear that their parents will learn about it.

14. What level of control should I have over my children's medical decisions as they approach and enter adolescence?

Most older children and adolescents are capable of understanding their various options for medical treatment. Therefore, depending upon the seriousness of their medical condition, the level of involvement they wish to have, their maturity level, and the needs of their family, adolescents should be encouraged to participate actively in the healthcare decision-making process.[8] Since adolescent patients are usually capable of understanding the risks and benefits of proposed treatments/procedures and their alternatives, their consent for medical interventions should also be obtained.

Most state laws indicate, however, that for the purposes of medical care a minor (person under "legal age," which varies from state to state) may not provide legally recognized informed consent for the performance of a medical or surgical procedure; rather, the consent of a parent or guardian is required. The exceptions to this involve instances in which emergency medical care is required, instances in which one or both parents may be unavailable to provide consent, or if certain other conditions apply. These conditions vary between jurisdictions, but some examples follow:

1. The minor is emancipated (no longer under his or her parents' authority), married, or homeless.
2. The proposed care is related to sexually transmitted diseases (STDs).
3. The proposed care is related to sexual assault or rape, and the minor is over twelve years of age.
4. The proposed care is related to alcoholism.
5. The proposed care is related to substance abuse.
6. The proposed care is related to testing for HIV (the virus that causes AIDS).

Abortion presents a unique situation. State-specific statutes must be consulted in cases in which a minor female requests an abortion. Laws requiring parental notification and/or consent prior to the performance of an abortion upon a minor are in effect in the vast majority of states (forty-three as of this writing). In cases in which the validity of federal or state laws is in question, the courts may become involved and determine whether/how the laws should be applied.

Although by law parents are typically required to give consent for their minor children's medical procedures and treatment, medical decision-making should, nevertheless, allow for input from the minor if he or she is developmentally able to offer it—especially in circumstances where lengthy and challenging procedures or treatments are required. It's clear that *compliance* issues might pose a major obstacle to successful treatment delivery if a child is unwilling to accept a certain medical intervention. While a child's resistance may not be overly problematic if directed toward procedures such as immunization (since parents routinely ignore their children's wishes in such instances and, if necessary, may even assist the physician in physically restraining the child so that shots may be administered), unwillingness becomes more significant in cases where lengthy and difficult medical treatments are needed. Consider the case of an adolescent who has failed to respond to treatment for cancer. A decision to try experimental therapy instead of opting for comfort care should take into account not only the parents' input, but also the patient's desires.

Ultimately, parents have medical decision-making authority over their children and should make decisions for their children based upon their overall good. Conflicts may arise in some situations, however, as to what constitutes such good. The case of a child or adolescent who is a Jehovah's Witness and requires a blood transfusion is one such example. If the patient desires to have the transfusion but his parents object, the physician should consider going to court in an attempt to have the patient's wishes respected. If, however, both the patient and her parents wish to forego the transfusion, the situation is more difficult. Respecting religious beliefs is, after all, an important part of respecting human dignity. A strong judicial precedent has, nevertheless, been established, allowing medical authorities to obtain a court order for transfusion in such situations. Ignoring this precedent and allowing a child or adolescent to die could have serious repercussions for the physician and possibly for the parents. Therefore, if the physician and/or parents deem that withholding transfusion is in the patient's best interests, he or they should petition the appropriate court for "judicial relief," i.e., the court's permission not to provide the transfusion.

15. What is the role of an ethics committee in a hospital or other healthcare institution?

The precise role of an ethics committee will vary depending upon the institution or organization within which it functions. Long-term care facilities, health maintenance organizations (HMOs), medical schools, community clinics, and hospice organizations may all have ethics committees. Additionally, biotechnology firms and state and federal authorities may have ethics committees. In general, though, the primary function of an ethics committee is to assist the patient, family, medical staff, and society in addressing the often complex ethical questions that arise in the context of medical decision-making. Most ethics committees are typically involved in bedside consultations, policy guidance, and education of medical staff and the community. The focus of a particular ethics committee will depend upon the experience of its members, how long the committee has been in existence, and the needs and resources of the institution or organization.

In bedside consultations, the interests and desires of the patient are primary, but other factors must be taken into account in determining the course of action that the committee will recommend. Patients may desire, for instance, that their doctors administer certain therapies or interventions that are either illegal or unethical. In such a case, the ethics committee should refuse to support the inappropriate request (see also questions 16–17).

Ethics committees do not generally set hospital policy. Hospital medical staffs are instead responsible for providing input to the hospital's board of trustees, which possesses ultimate authority regarding what policies are adopted. Most ethics committees do, however, propose new policies and initiate the process of review and (if necessary) revision of existing policies. The hospital's medical executive committee may also request that the ethics committee draft policy statements for review and consideration. If approved, the statements would then require approval by the board of trustees prior to implementation. In most cases, "Do Not Resuscitate" (DNR), discontinuation of treatment, advance directive, and many other policies are reviewed extensively by the hospital ethics committee prior to submission to the board of trustees for full approval and implementation.

Ethics committees also frequently focus on providing ethics education to medical staff and community members. These efforts may include making hospital rounds with staff members, participating in "grand rounds" discussions, giving lectures, preparing articles for publication in in-house journals, and/or leading or contributing to small-group discussions regarding particular bedside consultations. On occasion, ethics committee members may also help educate the wider community through various symposia or television appearances.

Most mid- to large-sized hospitals now have ethics committees. The Joint Commission on Accreditation of Healthcare Organizations (JCAHO) requires that in order for a hospital to receive JCAHO accreditation, a system must be in place for addressing patients' and families' ethical concerns. Those who have such concerns should check with their physician, the head administrative nurse on the hospital floor, or the hospital's administration office. In situations where a formal ethics committee or consultation team (see question 16) is not available, a parallel, similar method for resolving these concerns will typically be offered.

David Schiedermayer, M.D. and John La Puma, M.D. have coauthored a book entitled *Ethics Consultation: A Practical Guide* (Jones and Bartlett Publishers, Boston, 1994), which can serve as an excellent tool for those desiring to organize an ethics committee in their healthcare institution. Additionally, the Medical College of Wisconsin offers an Internet-based forum that addresses many of the commonly asked questions about ethics committees. The forum may be accessed at www.mcw.edu/bioethics.

16. What is an ethics consultation (or "consult"), and how can I arrange for one?

In most institutions, it would be too difficult to schedule a meeting of the whole ethics committee to discuss a patient situation for which decisions must be made quickly. Accordingly, some institutions have, in addition to an ethics committee, another body or subcommittee—called an *ethics consultation team*—that deals exclusively with ongoing patient-related ethical dilemmas.

An ethics consultation team is typically responsible for doing the "bedside work" related to consults. This might include interviewing the patient, meeting with the family, speaking with nurses and physicians, and identifying clearly the specific ethical issue(s) of concern. After thoughtful reflection, discussion, any further consultation, and, in some instances, full case review by the ethics committee, the consultation team will provide those who requested the consult with guidance and recommendations.

In some institutions, any member of the ethics committee might also function as a member of the ethics consultation team. In other settings, the consultation team may be a separate, smaller group with a particular interest and training in performing consultations. In yet other contexts, the consultations may be performed exclusively by one expert or by a few designated experts. Regardless of the particular approach, consults are usually reviewed at some point by the larger ethics committee. The remainder of this question will address a team approach.

In various healthcare institutions, different people are empowered to call for an ethics consultation. Usually the consultation is initiated at the request of a patient, family member, or any member of the healthcare team (e.g., nurse, social worker, chaplain, therapist, or physician). As noted in the previous answer, such requests should be made to the physician overseeing the case, the head administrative nurse (on a patient's hospital floor), or the institution's administration office. Those who make the request will be grappling with a specific question, such as "Is it ethical to discontinue life support for this dying patient?" or "Is the proposed course of action about to be taken ethical?" or "Is this treatment plan consistent with existing hospital ethics guidelines?"

When the consult team representative initially arrives to begin the exploratory phase of the consult, he or she will typically meet with the patient, healthcare professionals, and family members, if appropriate. The representative will help to determine if the issue is truly an ethical concern (as opposed to, for example, an administrative concern or one requiring legal guidance). If the concern is not truly an ethical one, it will be referred to the appropriate person(s), such as a nursing administrator, hospital attorney, chaplain, or social worker. If, on the other hand, it appears that the issue is appropriate for the consult team to address, a more extensive investigation will move forward.

The team will then evaluate the specific question in light of existing law, hospital policy, and intra-family and intra-team communication. Informal and (if need be) formal meetings may be held with the patient, the family, the treatment team, and perhaps other parties that the patient or family request be involved. These may include the family's pastor or, in certain settings, official representatives of the government (such as representatives from the Office of State Guardian or similar authorities). An amicable solution can most often be achieved, with the expressed concern(s) being addressed in a manner that is satisfactory to all involved. At other times, if no mutually acceptable decision can be reached, external arbitration, possibly at times involving the court system, may be necessary.

Most ethics consultation teams strive to be multi-disciplinary, utilizing chaplains, social workers, nurses, and perhaps others, along with physician representation. The multi-disciplinary nature of ethics consultation teams makes them especially well-equipped to address certain concerns that require more than a single perspective in order for the best resolution to be reached.

For more information, see the resources noted at the end of the previous question. In addition, the American Society of Bioethics and Humanities (ASBH) has created a helpful report, "Core Competencies for Health Care Consultation," which provides a good overview of basic elements of the ethics consultation, as well as suggestions for providing quality consultations. This resource is available from ASBH by calling (847) 375-4745 or by e-mailing info@asbh.org. The ASBH's Web site may be accessed at www.asbh.org.

17. How do ethics committees and consultants make ethical judgments, and how much authority do they have?

Ethics committees and consultants need some basis for determining whether the situations they are reviewing are ethical or unethical. Patients, families, and healthcare professionals also often need help in determining the best course of action.

No single ethical system has been adopted as the national standard for making healthcare decisions. Rather, many ethics committees and consultants endorse an ethical system adopted by their institution or, in some cases, one proposed by a persuasive member. As is true for most other committees, politics and social interplay will often affect the decision-making process. In addition, local laws, local traditions, and precedent all may serve to influence the decisions that are made. A Roman Catholic hospital, a secular university hospital, and a small rural hospital in Utah may, for example, hold to markedly different worldviews and ethical systems.

Nevertheless, Tom Beauchamp and James Childress have proposed an ethical system that has been widely embraced as a guide for healthcare decision-making. This system emphasizes four principles: *autonomy, beneficence, non-maleficence,* and *justice*. This model provides a common framework for ethical debate among people whose belief systems vary. The principle of *autonomy* is often emphasized, with the patient's wishes taking precedence as much as possible provided that laws and policies are not broken. *Beneficence* encompasses the importance of promoting patient well-being, while *non-maleficence* is the closely-related principle of not causing harm. *Justice* addresses issues related to the fair distribution of limited resources, as well as treatment costs.

While most people would affirm that all four principles are important, debate arises when the principles come into conflict. A decision to do what a patient desires may, for example, be seen as promoting patient autonomy, but someone else may view that decision as harming the patient or others. The practical work of an ethics committee often centers around resolving such disagreements. Many, in fact, have argued that applying these four principles to a particular situation may be a useful conversation starter, but that many other considerations must be involved if an ethical assessment is to be satisfactory.[9]

Many ethics committee members regard virtue, social benefit, or their own religious beliefs as the best guide to decision-making. Since ethics committees exist within a pluralistic society, however, the worldviews of individual committee members may not be given precedence. This pluralism can create dilemmas for Christian members, who want to influence the committee's decisions but may find themselves in a minority on the committee. Many ethics committees see their primary role as facilitating the wishes of patients, within the bounds of the law, which may further restrict the expression of the beliefs of individual committee members. Thus, membership on ethics committees can involve delicate and difficult interactions between people with different worldviews, requiring much sensitivity and wisdom. Various resources are available to help Christians undertake this task.[10]

In most states, an ethics committee or ethics consultation team's input is advisory only. Their function is primarily to help others make ethically sound decisions, not to make such decisions for them. This approach helps to preserve the centrality of the physician-patient relationship and prevents ethics committees and consultants from making decisions on medical matters for which they lack sufficient expertise. If, however, an ethics committee or consultation team discovers that a physician or medical team is proposing an intervention that they deem to be unethical, illegal, or otherwise improper, members of the ethics group are obligated to relay such information to a department head, chief of staff, vice-president of medical affairs, director of nursing, or other appropriate professional.

Although ethics committees or consultation teams function primarily in an advisory role, the possibility remains that their recommendations may occasionally involve a conflict of interest between the patient and the healthcare institution. To prevent this, the funding of such committees and teams should preferably not be controlled by those who stand to be most affected by the possible financial ramifications of ethics committee members' and consultants' decisions. Ethics committee and consultation team members should never feel that their continued participation in the ethics review process rests on whether their decisions will financially benefit the hospital or other healthcare organization involved.

ACCESS TO HEALTHCARE

---

18. Does everyone have a right to healthcare?

To answer this question, we must be clear about what is meant by a "right." This term is used frequently, but in very different ways. Rights can be based either in the law or in morals.

Legal rights are those that arise as a result of the Constitution or federal or state laws. Where there is a legal right, someone may be entitled to receive something, which others then have a duty to provide. Children have a right, for example, to a public education. Legal rights can also protect people from intrusion by the state. The government may not normally interfere, for instance, with free speech. In addition, legal rights may permit a person to forego a certain service or intervention. A patient has the legal right, for example, to refuse a medical treatment, based upon the underlying right of bodily integrity. This means that a doctor has a duty not to force or deceive a patient into accepting any treatment (see question 8). Doctors who violate this duty have violated the law.

Moral rights are not necessarily based upon the law of the land, although many moral rights are explicitly protected by law. Moral rights are founded on ethical principles concerning how best to treat others. Moral rights are usually one of two general types. The first, *liberty* (or negative) *rights* are based upon the idea that people have a right to be left alone to pursue their legitimate interests. The moral right to autonomy—that people can make their own decisions about their own healthcare—underlies the legal right to refuse treatment. (This legal right is also based on traditional protections against assault—an unwanted touching of one's body.) The moral right to privacy was one of the Supreme Court's justifications for legalizing abortion in the U.S. Liberty rights have come to dominate secular healthcare ethics in the U.S.

The second group of moral rights consists of what are called *entitlement* (or positive) *rights*. These are usually based more on one's view of justice. This approach to rights claims that people are unable to pursue their legitimate interests unless society supplies them with certain standard provisions. Entitlement rights are asserted in pursuit of a "level playing field" in the game of life. Such rights entitle people to receive certain basic social goods, such as education, police protection, and, some would argue, healthcare. An important aspect of these rights is that they always imply a corresponding duty. If people have a right to receive healthcare, then someone has a duty to provide that care. This inevitably raises the question, "Who will pay for the healthcare?" Another question that must also be addressed is, "What level of healthcare do people have a right to receive?" Does a person have the right to all the healthcare they might ever need or only to a certain level?

The World Health Organization (WHO) has stated clearly that, "The enjoyment of the highest attainable standard of health is one of the fundamental rights of every human being without distinction of race, religion, political belief, economic or social conditions." Given the huge disparity in the health standards of different countries around the world, most nations apparently do not take this "right" very seriously. Several countries have established a legal right entitling their citizens to receive a minimal standard of healthcare. In those countries, every citizen is guaranteed access to at least some level of healthcare.

The United States has not taken this approach. Healthcare is an entitlement right only for the elderly, the poor, and some disabled persons, and it is paid for through governmental Medicare and Medicaid programs. For most people in the U.S., though, healthcare falls under liberty rights: people are free to pursue whatever form of healthcare they desire, but they are not guaranteed to receive the healthcare they seek. Hence, people may choose to purchase health insurance, but they don't have a right to receive health insurance. This situation leaves many people questioning the U.S.'s commitment to justice, since more than 40 million citizens are without health insurance (largely because they can't afford it).

From a Christian perspective, discussions over rights often lead in the wrong direction, encouraging self-promotion. Christians are called to be concerned about the needs of poor persons in addition to their own (Prov. 29:7). Paul acknowledged that, as a Christian worker, he had a right to receive at least enough wages to feed himself (1 Cor. 9; 2 Thess. 3:7–9); yet he chose to give up this right to benefit others. In doing so, he followed the example that Jesus Christ put forward to guide all Christians in their actions: "Do nothing from selfishness or empty conceit, but with humility of mind let each of you regard one another as more important than himself; do not merely look out for your own personal interests, but also for the interests of others" (Phil. 2:3–4).

Our concern as Christians, then, should be for the rights of others and not just for our own rights. This mindset should also lead to a balanced perspective on how much healthcare we feel entitled to receive. We should be grateful for whatever healthcare resources we have, and when something isn't available or affordable, we should remain grateful for that which we've already received. We should not insist upon a right to all levels of healthcare, but only to a level that is socially equitable and affordable.

The United States is a very rich country with many more resources than most of the rest of the world. We begin with a standard of healthcare that is far beyond that experienced by people in many parts of the world. Yet even within the U.S., the distribution of healthcare is inequitable. God is deeply concerned about the welfare of those who are poor, and Christians should be also. Jesus came to this earth to give people life, true life (John 10:10). To the extent that bestowing upon people the right to healthcare will lead to a more just distribution of healthcare resources, Christians can support such an effort. That may require us to give up some of our other rights, such as an unlimited liberty right to acquire personal affluence. Such sacrifices would indeed appear to be very much in keeping with Jesus' sacrifice for us on the cross (Phil. 2:8).

19. Is it ethical to ration healthcare?

Rationing is the process of limiting the quantity of provisions (e.g., food, medicine, etc.) that will be made available to people. Rationing is necessary when there is a limited supply of a commodity that is basic to human needs. For example, food and fuel are often rationed during war-time. The notion of rationing usually suggests that the resources provided will be at least somewhat less than adequate. The possibility of rationing healthcare raises concerns that people will be told which healthcare resources they can and cannot have and that they may not be able to receive all the care they might need. For many people, rationing of healthcare does not seem ethical.

Food rationing during war-time is often required to ensure that everyone has access to an equal supply of the limited food available. If the food was not rationed but the supply was limited, prices might increase to the point where only the rich could afford to buy whatever was available. Rationing is, therefore, an attempt to apply principles of justice to the distribution of limited resources, guaranteeing all people a fixed amount of food by imposing restrictions on everyone. It is an attempt to prevent the rich and powerful from monopolizing the food supply at the expense of the poor and vulnerable. At its core, then, rationing is an ethical endeavor.

It may not be difficult to see the morality of rationing when a nation is at war. Most people recognize in such a situation that the nation must band together and make sacrifices so that the war can be won. It may be more difficult, though, to accept the application of rationing principles to healthcare systems during times of peace, as people may question what cause requires them to sacrifice for the good of others.

One of the healthcare myths that was shattered during the 1990s was the idea that everyone's healthcare costs could always be absorbed by "the system." Many people had assumed that as long as they had healthcare coverage through their job or paid their insurance premiums, whatever healthcare they needed would be available. As healthcare became increasingly technological and more costly treatments continued to be developed, the costs of providing healthcare grew astronomically. Although people naturally desired unlimited access to the best treatments available at a reasonable price, some limitations had to be put in place. While numerous solutions were proposed, the one that seemed most practical involved some degree of rationing. People would have to be told that they couldn't have access to whatever healthcare they wanted—unless they were able to pay for it with their own money.

To be ethical, rationing must be just. Although people differ in their ideas of what constitutes a just distribution of limited resources, justice would seem to require that everyone have access to at least the basic necessities of healthcare, much as war-time rations are designed to provide everyone with a basic level of nutrition.

Rationing healthcare differs from the rationing of other resources in that a person's need should influence what he receives. If everyone was given a fixed dollar value for healthcare each year, some people might not need this amount, while others who became ill or had an accident would need extra funds. Healthcare rationing must therefore allow for the sort of variability in need that comes with the uncertainties of life. The rationing of healthcare raises other complex issues, such as who will receive a scarce treatment and who will not. For rationing to be ethical, these decisions should be based upon objective criteria— such as the seriousness of a patient's condition and the willingness of the patient to receive the treatment in question. Rationing should not involve valuing people according to their contribution to society or permit the allocation of healthcare resources based upon prejudices. The inherent value and dignity of each individual must always be upheld, even while difficult resource allocation decisions are being made.

The arena of organ donation offers one of the clearest situations in which healthcare rationing occurs today. There are far more patients awaiting organ transplants than there are available organs. When a needed organ becomes available, a set of criteria is used to determine who will receive it. While these criteria are somewhat controversial, the goal is to make the selection process as objective as possible and to avoid any subjective bias that could influence decision-making.

The rationing of donated organs could be resolved if more organs were available. This would require the willingness of more people to serve as organ donors and the willingness of more families to allow the donations. If someone has expressed a desire to be an organ donor, this request should be upheld by the family, even though doing so may be difficult in the midst of the loved one's death. The organ donation can be one last gift that the deceased person can give to others who are in need.

The difficulties and undesirability of rationing should, then, motivate people to do everything ethically possible to increase the overall supply of healthcare resources.

Many medical conditions requiring costly treatments are, for instance, linked to lifestyle factors such as diet, exercise, and stress. If people would find ways to improve their health through lifestyle changes, the need for costly healthcare interventions would likely be reduced. These reduced expenses would translate into a greater availability of funds to treat other conditions.

Whenever individualism is held in high value, as it is in the United States, rationing will be unpopular. People like to be assured that they will receive all the care they need when they are ill. They must remember, however, that they're not just asking for healthcare, but are usually expecting others to pay for that care. In a perfect world, all people would have access to every resource they need. But such is not the case in our fallen world—even when it comes to healthcare. Given this truth, we should work to ensure that all rationing is done justly, distributing our available healthcare resources as wisely and as fairly as possible.

20. What sort of medical information is available on the Internet?

The Internet has rapidly become an integral part of daily life. Many people use e-mail to communicate at work and at home. Students of all ages use the Internet to conduct research for their school projects and papers. More and more consumers are searching for on-line product reviews before making purchases. It should be no surprise, then, that the Internet is also becoming a popular place to access medical information. According to a Harris Poll study, more than 100 million Americans use the Internet each year to find information—including health information.[11] Such popularity is reflected by the growing number of hospitals, healthcare facilities, and even individual doctors' offices that have Web sites designed to attract and inform people seeking to boost their knowledge about health issues.

The Internet is in many ways an attractive option for those pursuing medical and health information. Access is available twenty-four hours a day, seven days a week. All that is needed is a network-connected computer (which is available at many public libraries for those who don't have one at home, making accessibility affordable). Answers can be obtained quickly, and people can search out information in private without having embarrassing or awkward conversations with doctors or others who might ask why a person is seeking particular medical knowledge.

The Internet has great potential to help educate those who desire to take their health seriously. People can learn ways to make their lifestyles healthier and/or obtain information about a particular disorder that they or their loved ones may have. They can also contact individuals with whom they share medical conditions and experiences and thus establish "cyber-support groups." In addition, they may locate doctors in their vicinity (or anywhere else), as well as research or support organizations dedicated to a particular disease or disability who can best help them address their healthcare needs.

All of these potential benefits, however, can turn into liabilities because of the overarching problem that plagues every area of the Internet: the quality of what gets published is not monitored. When people without medical training turn to the Internet (or to any other published source of medical information) for health advice, they may not have the knowledge needed to evaluate the accuracy of that information.

In its May 23, 2001, issue, the *Journal of the American Medical Association (JAMA)* published a helpful study on the quality of medical information found on the Internet.[12]

The study examined the most popularly used medical Web sites and found them to be readily accessible, with important information relatively easy to locate. Eighty to ninety percent of the information found on all Web sites was determined to be accurate, with only a small percentage of the material reported as being completely inaccurate. In one-third of the sites reviewed, however, contradictions were found in recommendations for treatment. This discrepancy led the researchers to worry that people might come away from their Internet searches more confused than enlightened.

The *JAMA* study revealed another problem concerning the completeness of information on the Internet. A panel of experts developed a list of important topics that a patient should learn about when searching for information on a specific medical condition. Most of the English language Web sites for these medical conditions barely managed to mention half of these topics, and Spanish Web sites mentioned less than half of these topics. Moreover, the information was typically written at a high reading level. The average reading level of material on Spanish Web sites was tenth grade, while material on English sites was generally presented at the collegiate level—with one in ten of these Web sites written at the graduate school level. Such reading levels would make it difficult for almost half of the United States population—especially those who are poor and not well educated—to understand the information.

The *JAMA* study suggests another caution to keep in mind as one searches the Internet for medical information. While the results regarding the accuracy of the information were encouraging, this research focused only on the most popular Web sites. Great variability is found in the accuracy of the information available on other sites. The most accurate Web sites are those that are run by professional or governmental organizations or that employ properly trained and experienced experts to write their content. Before relying upon information from a Web site, find out who is sponsoring or funding the Web site. If this isn't easy to determine, be cautious. When evaluating a particular product or service, beware of Web sites that sell the products or services they describe. Some sites can resist the conflict of interest, but it's always important to compare their advice with Web sites known to be unbiased. Web sites selling drugs, herbal remedies, dietary supplements, or unconventional diagnostic tools are particularly prone to much variability of information.

Regardless of what medical advice you find on the Internet, it is crucial that you talk with your healthcare professionals before making major changes in your diet or lifestyle and/or before taking any drugs, vitamins, supplements, or herbs you read about on-line. Ask your healthcare professionals about the Web sites they use and why they recommend them. While the Internet offers many benefits, remember that its advice is always general. While much can be learned from the Internet, healthcare professionals are still indispensable in helping people to evaluate their personal medical conditions and to determine the best course of action for preventing illness or promoting recovery.

21. If I have faith in God, should I still seek a physician's care for medical problems?

An often-told story tells about a devout Christian man who was stranded on a desert island. The man prayed and prayed that God would rescue him. He knew he was asking for a miracle, but he never despaired—such was the strength of his faith. One morning he awoke to the sound of human voices! He ran to the shore, startling the crew of a small sailing boat anchored just off the island. The crew sent a boat over to the island and invited the stranded man to come aboard. They offered to take him to a port from where he could make his way home. The man thought, prayed silently, and then said, "No thank you. I know my God will rescue me Himself." The crew reluctantly set sail, leaving the man on his knees, deep in prayer. "What strong faith!" the captain remarked. Many days went by. The man saw no other boats, and his food and water supply ran out. Still, he never lost confidence in God. Then he died.

When the man arrived in heaven, God seemed a little upset. "What were you thinking down there?" God asked. "I trusted you, God," the man replied. "I believed you would rescue me. Why didn't you save me from dying on that island?" God looked at the man with pity and asked, "Who do you think sent that boat to anchor off your island?"[13]

We live in a world that often views God's activities as separate from the actions of human beings or nature. If we see a person's health restored following a medical procedure, we may fail to attribute any aspect of the healing to God. When we see a beautiful flower, we often fail to attribute its magnificence to anything more than the laws of nature and therefore don't give the glory to God, Who created flowers. Most of us have a weak perception of what theologians call the "sovereignty of God." Such a perception, though, does not stem from the picture of God that we are given in the Bible. When, for instance, Joseph's brothers sold him into slavery, he could have looked at his situation through purely human eyes. But instead, he saw that God was at work to bring about good even in his siblings' treachery (Gen. 45:4–7).

As Christians, we can rejoice in the direct supernatural care of God, as well as in the care He brings through others. One of the ways God cares for human beings is by empowering people to serve one another and to help those who are sick. This may involve demonstrating general care and concern, but may also include the administration and application of various remedies and technologies. Physicians are generally viewed very positively in the Bible (Jer. 8:22; Luke 4:23; Col. 4:14). Scripture also includes accounts of people cleansing, bandaging, and soothing wounds with oil (Isa. 1:5–6; James 5:14) or balm (Jer. 8:22) and setting fractures (Ezek. 30:21). Such was the medical care of that day. Medicine can, indeed, be a means by which God provides for people, just as are food, water, and shelter.

The value God places on health should not, however, be seen as a license or requirement to pursue any and all medical interventions. Difficult decisions must sometimes be made about when to withhold or withdraw a therapy that is of no benefit to, or is excessively burdensome for, a patient (see the *End of Life Decisions* booklet in this series). Although death is indeed an enemy (1 Cor. 15:26) and should never be intentionally caused by human beings, there are nevertheless situations in which it should not be resisted at any cost. Scripture also teaches that Christians should avoid therapies that are intimately intertwined with non-Christian religious ideas (see the *Alternative Medicine* booklet in this series), as God instructed the Israelites to avoid the pagan healers around them (2 Kings 1:2–4; 2 Chron. 16:12).

In general, the care of physicians—and the medicines they recommend—should be seen as part of God's provision for those who are ill or injured. Although some medical therapies will be inappropriate for Christians and there is the potential for any medical intervention to be misused or substituted for God in a person's life, we should be thankful for the medical resources we have and use them to the extent that's ethically appropriate.

22. Is it okay for me to make use of medical treatments that result from unethical research or procedures?

This question arises in part because people can be legally guilty of a crime even without directly participating in the actual criminal act. It's a crime, for instance, to knowingly receive stolen property obtained from a theft committed by someone else. During World War II, horrific medical experiments were carried out on prisoners in the Nazi concentration camps. Following the war, a debate erupted as to whether the results of this research should ever be used as a means of furthering medicine. Did the inhumane way the experiments were conducted so taint the data that any application of such would itself also be tainted? What if useful information that might save lives could be gained from the research? Would using this data further disrespect the victims, or would it bring some good from otherwise terrible circumstances?

The dilemma of the Nazi situation was largely resolved by a 1990 article in *The New England Journal of Medicine*.[14] A historical review found that the remaining Nazi data (much of it was destroyed by the Nazis themselves) is so scientifically flawed that it is worthless. The author marveled that such bad science had become the center of fifty years of ethical debate. The general question, though, remains: Is it acceptable to make use of the fruits of unethical research? This question will likely become more and more pressing, especially for Christians. As medical researchers increasingly carry out experiments relying upon human embryos, fetal tissue, and controversial genetic procedures, patients may be offered medical treatments developed from what many would view as unethical procedures. What principles should guide our decisions as to whether or not to make use of such treatments?

While we certainly empathize with people who have a

serious illness or debilitating injury, the praiseworthy end of alleviating illness and suffering does not justify all means. Christians should enthusiastically support the development of medical therapies from non-embryonic stem cell research and other methods that do not require the destruction of human beings.[15] While most Christians and others who uphold the dignity of all human life (including embryos) would agree with the above statement, the question remains as to whether it is acceptable to make use of medical treatments derived from unethical research or procedures that have been carried out *in the past*. That is, while there is a consensus among these communities that human embryos should not be destroyed for the purpose of furthering medical research, no such consensus exists as to whether it is ethical to conduct such research using embryos who have *already* been killed. Following President Bush's August 9, 2001, announcement of his decision that federal funds may be used to support only embryonic stem cell research involving embryos who had already been destroyed, Christian and pro-life groups were atypically divided in their reactions.

The President believed that his decision was consistent with his earlier campaign promise not to allow federal funding for stem cell research in which embryos are destroyed. By funding research only on cells derived from embryos for whom "the life-and-death decision has already been made,"[16] Bush contended that he was simultaneously objecting to the act of destroying embryos. Indeed, the President refused to allot funding for research requiring future embryonic destruction. Some, though, have questioned whether the government can fund *any* embryonic stem cell research and truly remain innocent. They ask whether the government is complicit in the evil of destroying human life by supporting research dependent upon such destruction.

In addressing this dilemma, an important question must be considered: Is it just the destruction of human embryos that should be opposed, or should research *dependent upon such destruction* also be condemned? If an embryo has already been destroyed, can a person who objects to such an act support research on the embryo's stem cells and still be regarded as morally consistent? Or is supporting the research equivalent to supporting the necessary destruction of embryonic life? Answers to these questions must be obtained before we can answer the more general question as to whether it's acceptable to use medical treatments that result from unethical research or procedures.[17]

Another controversial situation involves the use of certain vaccines that were developed using tissue obtained from elective abortions. Some Christians and others who acknowledge the sanctity of all human life believe that these vaccines are morally tainted by the process that led to their development, while others believe that use of these vaccines is morally acceptable. Although similarly complex, this issue is distinct from the stem cell research issue in at least two important ways.

First, the use of these vaccines does not require further abortions, while the development and wide-scale use of embryonic stem cell therapies will almost certainly require the additional sacrifice of human embryos. Second, the decisions to have the two original abortions from which the vaccines were developed were made without any knowledge that the tissue would be used in research, and vaccine development probably does not impact abortion decisions today. In contrast, couples who donate their embryos to stem cell research do so with the full knowledge that they will be used (destroyed) for research purposes. These couples have, in fact, *chosen* this fate for their embryos over the options of embryo adoption by other couples or cryopreservation (storage for possible later implantation).[18]

It's fortunate that vaccines, the development of which did not involve aborted tissue, are available for immunizing against many diseases. We believe that Christians should use these alternatives whenever possible to avoid any appearance of condoning abortion. Vaccines for chicken pox, hepatitis A, and rubella (German measles), however, are not available in the United States in any other form. If people choose not to receive these vaccinations or not to have them administered to their children, many more people will become infected with these diseases. Since rubella infections in pregnant women can lead to serious birth defects and since our society increasingly encourages abortion of babies known to have such defects, not using the vaccine could lead to the tragic consequence of more abortions. While this possibility should be taken into account, anticipated—or even certain—benefits (in this case, the prevention of particular harms) are themselves not sufficient to justify the use of unethical means.

The above dilemmas are very complex and challenging. In a perfect world, researchers would be completely ethical in their work. However, we live in a fallen world, and some of the benefits we enjoy today are the result of earlier unethical acts. If we try to avoid anything that has the slightest moral taint, there would be little that we would not reject. Many of our country's current economic benefits can, for example, be traced back to unethical means of taking land from Native Americans and using African slaves to develop that land. Yet most of us do not regard these benefits as "tainted," but instead enjoy them.

Lapses in research ethics continue to occur today. In trying to bring a helpful treatment to market, researchers might, for instance, rush potential subjects into clinical studies, thereby violating the ethical pillar of medical research that subjects be truly informed of the research's potential benefits, risks, and alternatives. Since that research would then be regarded as unethical, should Christians avoid the resultant therapy? We believe that, while the breach of ethics should be denounced and efforts taken to prevent its recurrence, the treatment could still be used with good conscience. In such cases, it was the research methodology that was unethical, not the treatment itself. So long as the treatment is still supported by sufficient research that is both ethically and scientifically valid, Christians could make use of these products.

To be sure, life in a fallen world is not as it should be. To hold to the highest possible ethical standards requires a strict analysis of our own personal lives. How many of the current benefits we enjoy would God view as being tainted by selfish, unloving, or unethical origins? An honest appraisal should lead us to ask humbly for God's forgiveness for our sin, repent of our sinful ways, and seek discernment so that we may turn away from evil and toward good (Matt. 6:13; Heb. 5:12–14). We need to adopt a similar approach in our evaluation of medical research.

The answer to this question, then, is exceedingly complicated. If a treatment involves the repetition of an unethical act, it should not be used. If a treatment has any ethical taint due to the history of its development and an alternative can be used, or the treatment is not really necessary, it should be avoided. Such guidelines may also place pressure on researchers to be more ethical in the future.

Christians may not always reach the same conclusions regarding questions surrounding unethical research. Because "gray areas" do exist, we must make prayerful, informed decisions and adopt an attitude of hesitancy before speaking out against the actions of others.[19]

23. How safe are blood transfusions, and is it ethical to refuse them?

As noted in the answer to question 7 regarding informed consent, no treatment or procedure is without some degree of risk. Blood transfusions, therefore, are not risk-free. It is possible to contract AIDS or hepatitis or to suffer a negative reaction following receipt of a blood transfusion. Before consenting to a transfusion, then, it is important to consider the likelihood of these risks actually occurring.

Figures available from the American Association of Blood Banks (www.aabb.org/All_About_Blood/FAQs/ aabb_faqs.htm#6) quantify the various risks associated with blood transfusions as follows: The chance of developing AIDS from a blood transfusion is estimated to be less than 1 in 1.9 million for each unit of blood received. The number of patients who have developed AIDS as the result of a blood transfusion has dramatically decreased in recent years, especially since the introduction in 1999 of a new test (the nucleic acid test) to detect blood contamination. As even better tests become available, the chance of developing AIDS from a blood transfusion may, in the not too distant future, be reduced to near zero. Currently the risk of developing hepatitis B as the result of a blood transfusion is estimated to be 1 in 137,000, and the risk of becoming infected with hepatitis C through blood transfusion is approximately 1 in 1 million. In addition to the above risks, negative reactions to blood transfusions are possible. The two most serious reactions, which could be life-threatening, are known as *hemolytic transfusion reactions* and *anaphylactic reactions.* These reactions occur within a range of 1 in 20,000 to 1 in 50,000 blood transfusions. Although such reactions are sometimes life-threatening, most are not and respond well to medical treatment.

While this information may be helpful in making decisions about blood transfusions, a more general question about risk in medical treatment should be addressed: "As a Christian, what is my responsibility to accept medical therapies that carry risk of further harm in order to treat a health condition?" The answer isn't always simple. The best way to approach this problem is to weigh the benefits of the proposed therapy against its risks, a process that requires great discernment. God requires us to act in accordance with His will and not just in accordance with our own preferences, thus underscoring for Christians the importance of determining whether or not to receive a particular medical treatment.

In situations where the anticipated benefits of a treatment are great and the risks are minimal, it's easy to conclude that a patient should accept the treatment. We're expected to seek healing and avail ourselves of healthcare when it's available. Jesus spent much of His earthly ministry actively healing the sick, and God works through healthcare professionals today. To refuse medical care without sufficient reason is to reject God's plan for our lives.

In situations, though, where the proposed treatment is highly unlikely to prolong life but may increase suffering, it's relatively easy to conclude that any potential benefits are outweighed by the burdens of the treatment. This may be especially true of experimental therapies. While we don't wish to imply that it's wrong for a patient to request these therapies, we simply acknowledge that it may be morally permissible to refuse such treatment.

Situations also occur in which the benefits and risks of

a therapy are closely balanced. While decision-making in such cases may be difficult, Christians are generally urged to err on the side of preserving their lives and thus their continued ability to serve God. Still, such decisions require prayer, mature counsel, and great discernment.

In the particular case of blood transfusions, the overall risk of harm is very small and our current blood supply is now considered to be safer than at any time in the past. For this reason, assuming that a transfusion is expected to have a positive or even life-saving effect, it should typically be received.

24. Should I pursue only treatments that are medically necessary, or is it okay for me to pursue those that will simply enhance my quality of life?

This question assumes that Christians should pursue medically necessary treatments. Medicine provides one way by which Christians can maintain their health or treat illness. Paul reminded the Corinthian Christians, "Do you not know that your body is a temple of the Holy Spirit, who is in you, whom you have received from God? You are not your own; you were bought at a price. Therefore honor God with your body" (1 Cor. 6:19–20). Medically necessary treatments often enable people to be good stewards of the lives and bodies with which they have been blessed. Christians, however, are not always required to pursue all available medical treatments. The question of when medical treatment can be foregone or withdrawn is addressed in detail in the *End of Life Decisions* booklet of this series.

Advances in medical science have led to the development of many new products. Some treat or prevent conditions such as baldness or wrinkled skin, which would not traditionally be regarded as illnesses. Other medications provide important medical benefits for people with certain conditions, but may also be used simply as a way to enhance quality of life. Human growth hormone (hGH) is an example of such a medication. Some people produce subnormal quantities of this hormone and therefore take supplements, much like diabetic patients take insulin. Such a use of hGH is entirely appropriate. This hormone is sometimes given, however, to shorter-than-average children who have completely normal hormone levels in order to help these children grow taller, thereby sparing them some of the embarrassment and discrimination associated with being short. Viagra, Prozac, and Ritalin are other drugs that have legitimate medical uses but are sometimes used in the absence of medical necessity as a means to improve quality of life. Genetic research is likely to further increase the availability of such "quality of life" treatments.

Should treatments that are not medically necessary be employed solely for the purpose of improving quality of life? In answering this question, we'll consider the condition of baldness. Baldness, to the best of our knowledge, carries no health risks in itself. Some people, though, do not want to be bald and may even feel bad about being bald. They may have fewer opportunities for dating and marriage and may even be discriminated against in their careers. These feelings and experiences may lead to depression, anxiety, and lowered self-esteem. Could there be any problem with taking a pill that might prevent or reverse baldness, thereby eliminating these negative psychological effects?

In responding to this question, one must first consider issues of safety and effectiveness. As stated, baldness itself does not carry any inherent health risks. All medical treatments, on the other hand, carry some risk of side effects, especially medications that might need to be taken for extended periods of time. The risk of those side effects may be relatively high and may not be worth assuming, especially if the chances of successful treatment are relatively low. People should carefully investigate the safety and efficacy of quality-of-life treatments especially when the health risks of not treating a particular condition are negligible or non-existent.

Many people claim that they should have the right to take whatever medications they desire, provided they can afford to pay for them. People *do* have this right today in America. There's nothing inherently wrong with trying to change one's hairline, height, or quality of life. Christians, though, should always consider more than just their personal autonomy and the inherent wrongness of an action. In the context of making decisions regarding non-moral issues, Paul reminds us, "'Everything is permissible'—but not everything is beneficial. 'Everything is permissible'—but not everything is constructive. Nobody should seek his own good, but the good of others" (1 Cor. 10:23–24). Even if we have the personal freedom to choose treatments that are not medically necessary, Christians should reflect upon how choosing to take certain medications might impact others. The negative effects of baldness mentioned above stem from people's *responses* to baldness. The bald person may, for instance, feel bad about being bald, or other people may treat the bald person badly. A Christian response should focus on how God can help people deal with their insecurities. A poor self-esteem is most effectively addressed by focusing on truths such as one's blessedness in the Lord and the fact that he or she is made in the image of God (Eph. 1), rather than by taking steps to remove or improve an undesired characteristic. Oftentimes, because such improvement or removal does not address the root issues behind people's insecurities, their self-esteem may remain poor following the intervention. Treatments that are not medically necessary tend to focus on the externals, while the roots of personal insecurities lie in people's hearts, which only God can fix (Matt. 15:18–20). The increasing popularity of treatments that are not medically necessary may, however, put more pressure on people to change externally, rather than to accept themselves and change internally.

Such treatments may also have a direct effect on others, more so than may be apparent. Important patterns are now being established with regard to the use of currently available medications that are not medically necessary. Decisions about taking these medications should be made in light of biblical principles concerning good stewardship. The money we spend is not ours, but God's (Ps. 24:1). When we pay for a treatment that is not medically necessary, that money is no longer available to meet the needs of others. "Each man should give what he has decided in his heart to give, not reluctantly or under compulsion, for God loves a cheerful giver" (2 Cor. 9:7). We should thus prayerfully consider these expenditures just as we should consider any other non-essential purchase. For the sake of upholding important principles, then, especially those of love and justice, Christians should be willing to deny themselves some of the apparent benefits of these medications.

On a larger scale, drug companies are making huge investments in—as well as profits from—products that are taken to enhance people's quality of life. While people in affluent nations spend billions on Viagra and Prozac for non-medical reasons, those in poorer nations have little or no healthcare or food. God is especially concerned about justice and the needs of the poor (Matt. 23:23). To paraphrase 1 John 3:17, how can the love of God be in those of us who are rich but who have no pity on those we know are in need? The choices made by those of us who are rich impact the amount of resources available to meet the basic needs of those who are starving and dying of treatable illnesses. We must, therefore, choose well, rather than simply choosing what we may desire.

FINANCING HEALTHCARE

25. What should I do if I can't afford health insurance?

To answer this question well, it is important first to consider the reasons why you are unable to afford health insurance. Some people's financial situations may be beyond their control. The apostle Paul called on the Church to care for those who, through no fault of their own, find themselves in financial need. In his day, widows were frequently poor due to neglect by their families and society in general. Paul called on the widows' Christian family members to care for them, and for the Church to provide any additional needed assistance (1 Tim. 5:3–9). People who are today unable to afford health insurance as a result of unavoidable hardship should likewise turn not only to the resources generally available in today's society, but also to their families and church families for possible help. The body of Christ is there, in large part, to help carry one another's burdens, which may include addressing spiritual and stewardship issues (Gal. 6:2).

While promoting care of the needy, Paul himself went to great lengths not to be a financial burden upon others. Although it may sound harsh, Paul declared that, "If a man will not work, he shall not eat" (2 Thess. 3:10). People who cannot afford health insurance because they refuse to work or because they've made unwise choices in their spending should assume responsibility for adjusting their habits so that insurance can be afforded. They should pray for wisdom to begin managing their affairs in ways that will glorify God, and ask others to pray for them as they seek to make necessary changes in their lives.

The Church should be committed to developing creative ways to help those who lack health insurance. Doctors, nurses, and other healthcare professionals within the Church may be able to provide healthcare at a reduced (or no) cost, allowing people without insurance to care for themselves and their families. Parish nurses can also play an important role here (see question 5). Other church members may be able to use their contacts in the community to help those in need find better jobs or pursue training that will allow them to afford health insurance. The Church might also be able to negotiate with health insurance companies so that they begin to offer programs providing some sort of coverage for those who can least afford it. For any of this to occur, the Church must become more than simply a group of Christians who meet once a week. The Church must become a community of people who are aware of the needs around them and who are concerned about all of its members. The Church is called to function as the body of Christ, which suffers when any member suffers (1 Cor. 12:22–26).

The local church may not be able to meet all needs, though. For example, many people with healthcare needs are not Christians or are not involved in a church. The Church should indeed seek to meet the needs of those outside its own community when possible, as it is more equipped to care for the whole person than are secular agencies. But when other resources are not available, government agencies in the United States exist to provide health insurance (e.g., Medicare and Medicaid) for those who truly cannot afford it or who have special needs. A helpful government Web site (www.ahcpr.gov/consumer/insuranc.htm) explains the differences between the many types of health insurance and government assistance available to help those without healthcare coverage. State and local agencies vary across the country and from one city to another, so listing all of them here is not possible. But by calling any local hospital or government agency, those in need should be able to obtain direction to resources within their communities where they can obtain the help and advice they seek.

Over forty million Americans are currently without health insurance, and this number is increasing. For many people, lack of insurance may not be a significant problem unless a medical catastrophe strikes. While everyone is at some risk for suffering a serious illness or injury, people who cannot afford health insurance may feel they simply have no choice but to forego coverage. With no health insurance, though, just one serious illness or accident could be enough to wipe out a person financially. The guidelines offered here are general, but are designed to help direct you toward resources should you or someone you know be unable to afford health insurance.

26. Is it ever ethical for my insurance company to refuse to cover treatments?

Most people living in the United States are used to having health insurance cover the majority of their medical expenses. When we become ill, we believe we should be able to receive whatever therapies or procedures we need to become well again. The idea that someone with a serious medical condition might die because he or she was denied coverage for treatment seems wrong to us. We believe that if we pay our insurance premiums we should be able to obtain whatever care we need.

We seem to forget, though, that health insurance companies are businesses that must operate according to sound financial principles. The health insurance system is basically a way of distributing healthcare costs so that more people can afford some level of care. All insurance programs, no matter what type they are, collect a certain amount of money in premiums to pay the healthcare expenses of those who are insured. While individuals may view their insurance as *"their* policy for meeting *their* needs,"* those who are insured are actually members of a community that help one another afford healthcare. While this community may not be visible to individual members, the premiums paid by each member, taken together, cover the members' medical expenses as well as whatever business administration costs are incurred and also yield the profit that the insurance company seeks.

Health insurance companies must balance their financial interests with their ethical responsibilities. Such companies have an ethical responsibility to manage wisely and justly the money entrusted to them. A company that generates huge profits or pays its executives exorbitant salaries by frequently denying its clients coverage for necessary treatments is operating unethically. A balance must be maintained between running the health insurance company as a business and realizing that what the company provides is a basic necessity, often with life-and-death implications.

In addition, those who are insured must make ethical decisions with regard to their healthcare pursuits. If every participant in a particular health insurance program insisted on having the costs of highly expensive (but unnecessary) treatments covered by the company, no one could afford the resulting premiums. Small organizations with their own insurance plans often see huge premium increases after only one member is involved in a serious accident or suffers a devastating illness. It is important, therefore, that persons do not make insurance claims for medical interventions that are not essential.

Given this understanding of insurance, we can envision situations in which it might be ethical for insurance companies to deny coverage for certain medical interventions. The motivation behind such coverage denials, however, should not be to increase profits or salaries for the insurance company. Rather, insurance companies may ethically refuse to cover certain treatments in order that the basic healthcare needs of everyone in the plan can be covered at a reasonable premium.

Insurance companies could, for instance, ethically refuse to cover treatments that it deems to be medically unnecessary. A person may desire a costly procedure to reduce the appearance of facial wrinkles, even though wrinkles will generally not lead to further medical problems. Such an intervention should be viewed as entirely optional, rather than medically necessary—if a person can afford it, she may make the decision to pursue it, but the cost of the procedure should not be spread among those who are insured.

Insurance coverage could also ethically be denied for treatments of questionable effectiveness. Insurance companies often do not cover experimental treatments because companies can provide the most benefit with limited funds by financing treatments with proven rather than unproven benefits. Meanwhile, new research sometimes reveals that treatments that have become standard practice are actually no more effective than placebos. On the other hand, research may reveal that a new and very expensive drug may, for most people, be no better than an older, less expensive drug. If an older drug would be completely adequate for meeting a particular patient's healthcare needs, the insurance company could ethically deny coverage of the new drug while offering to cover the cost of the older drug.

Another form of denial that may be ethical (although difficult to accept) is insurance companies' refusal to cover the cost of services administered by healthcare professionals who are not within their plan. In doing so, the insurance companies are seeking a balance between providing access to healthcare and operating according to business principles. Insurance companies sometimes arrange to direct their clients to certain healthcare professionals who have in turn agreed to charge fixed fees for their services. Such a practice might be ethical if motivated by the desire to provide affordable coverage for all who are insured within the plan. If, however, such an arrangement resulted in "kick-backs" (inappropriate financial rewards) for the healthcare professionals, it would be unethical. If the system resulted in limited access to competent healthcare professionals, it might also be unethical. The assumption is, however, that many healthcare professionals are able to provide adequate care for many conditions. While we may desire to see the very best specialist in the country for our particular medical concern, this may be neither necessary nor practical.

Insurance companies should inform their clients ahead of time about the types of treatments that will not be covered and should offer a sound rationale for such decisions. Clients (especially those who are Christians) should, on the other hand, understand that they are not just autonomous individuals, but that the healthcare decisions they make will have consequences for others. Although we may often fail to realize it, the members of an insurance plan are indeed interdependent.

We live in a world with limited resources. Those of us living in a country such as the United States, where access to healthcare is generally available, should be grateful. While we may be accustomed to having seemingly unlimited choices for everything from ice cream flavors to automobiles, much of the world is dying from starvation and a total lack of healthcare. Yet even in our plentiful environment, we must sometimes choose to put our good as individuals below the good of the many. Great wisdom and discernment is needed in making these sorts of decisions to ensure that they are just and otherwise ethical.

27. What should I do if my healthcare plan won't pay for a treatment I desire?

Finding out that your healthcare plan doesn't cover a desired medical treatment is often very disappointing. The answer to question 26 discussed why we believe health insurance companies can ethically refuse to cover particular types of interventions. Our focus here will be on how Christians ought to respond when told that their insurance will not pay for a certain treatment. Our discussion will be limited to situations in which treatments are not covered because the insurance company considers them to be cosmetic, experimental, or inappropriate.

When people are told that their healthcare plans will not pay for a desired treatment, it's normal for them to react emotionally. They may feel disappointed, frustrated, hurt, or angry. It is important that they recognize these feelings and discuss them with mature, trustworthy friends and family members before rushing too quickly to appeal such decisions.

Whenever a request for a particular treatment is refused, it is crucial to examine the motives behind the desire for that treatment. Remember the words of James in his New

Testament letter: "You do not have, because you do not ask God. When you ask, you do not receive, because you ask with wrong motives, that you may spend what you get on your pleasures" (James 4:2–3). In the context of medical care, it is important to carefully consider whether you desire a treatment that (medically speaking) you don't really need. The distinction between medical needs and non-medical desires is becoming more difficult to delineate as clinical treatments for conditions such as hair loss, shortness, and obesity are increasingly being offered. It's therefore all the more necessary to reflect carefully on the values and motives underlying your request. If you determine that you desire a treatment for non-medical reasons, you may need to accept a refusal of coverage and be grateful for the coverage that you have for other conditions.

Apart from the question of whether a treatment is being sought for medical or non-medical reasons, many insurance companies have decided that they will not cover drugs and procedures that are still being evaluated in research. The companies often cite a legitimate desire to protect those whom they insure from highly risky treatments. Although such an approach could keep some patients from receiving new and effective therapies, we must remember that experimental treatments, by definition, are unproven. Most are never marketed, either because they have been shown not to work or because they have too many side effects. If coverage for such a treatment is denied, it may be best to seek out other treatments of proven efficacy that your healthcare plan will cover or, when possible, to respond with patience. If the experimental treatment does become approved, it will most likely then be covered by insurance. If, though, your condition is so serious that a yet unapproved treatment is your only hope for recovery, you may be able to receive it by participating in the ongoing research designed to evaluate it. Other mechanisms for providing experimental treatments to people who have no other options may also be available. In such cases, the developer of a particular treatment will often help cover its cost. To learn more about these possibilities, talk to your physician or to the professional from whom you learned about the experimental treatment.

The final common reason that a healthcare plan may deny coverage is when a request for a treatment is determined to be inappropriate. One person may, for example, desire a therapy that has no known benefit for persons with his condition, while another may desire an expensive treatment even though she has only a very short time to live, regardless of the intervention administered. While such determinations are often legitimately made by physicians, they can sometimes be reinforced by a lack of health insurance coverage, forcing us to face the fact that we live in a fallen world.

Whether we are forced to endure the flu without antibiotics, adjust to a disability that can't be corrected, or face the inevitability of our death, we live in a world where suffering simply cannot always be avoided. There is not a pill for every ill. And just because we desire some particular treatment doesn't mean that it will help us or that we have an inherent right to obtain it.

If you evaluate your reasons for seeking a particular treatment and conclude that you have legitimate medical need for it but are denied coverage, your next step should be to begin the appeals process. Enlist the help of your physician and contact your insurance company, stating your case in writing as reasonably as possible. If you still fail to obtain coverage, you should then look into other ways to pay for the needed treatments, either through loans or grants. You might also consider approaching family members or people in your church for assistance. If your needs are indeed legitimate and significant, people will most likely want to help.

Throughout experiences like these you should, above all, seek the Lord, Who will ultimately comfort you in your time of need, and reflect upon Jesus Christ, Who accepted the fact that He would suffer and die on this earth. Similarly, the apostle Paul asked God to remove his thorn in the flesh, but God refused. From this, Paul learned to depend upon the Lord in deeper ways, declaring, "For when I am weak, then I am strong" (2 Cor. 12:10). Paul learned to be content, no matter what his circumstances (Phil. 4:11). So, too, can God help us accept the medical conditions we cannot change, including those for which treatment coverage is denied.

28. *What is managed care?*

Managed care is a form of *third party payment* or health insurance that integrates an insurance company's financial incentives with delivery of appropriate medical care. The major difference between managed care and traditional health insurance is that some of the financial risk of treating patients is assumed by the physician or group of physicians. The arena of managed care involves numerous terms that may be unfamiliar to many people. This answer will focus on defining these terms and may, therefore, seem somewhat abstract. The ensuing ethical issues raised by managed care will be addressed in the answer to question 29.

Direct *fee-for-service* has been the traditional method of payment for medical services. In this arrangement, a patient pays the physician or hospital for services rendered. A *sliding scale fee-for-service,* in which the amount of compensation is based upon a patient's ability to pay, may be another option. Initial judgments about a patient's ability to pay are made by the treating physician, and some physicians in private practice settings will occasionally decide to waive a patient's bill altogether. Some clinics who have either governmental, church, or private foundation support are also able to subsidize care and offer a discounted fee-for-service to needy patients, although health clinics and centers that currently offer a sliding scale fee-for-service usually require some documentation of the patient's financial status before adjusting the bill.

Third party payment of medical expenses is a relatively recent development. Health insurance funded by private companies or the government spreads the actual costs of healthcare over a large number of people, thereby keeping the costs for any individual relatively low. In the United States, people who receive health insurance through their employers are able to finance their healthcare coverage with pre-tax dollars, resulting in considerable savings for those who are insured in this way. The original purpose of third party payments was to offer an alternative way to pay fee-for-service bills.

In the last several decades, healthcare costs have soared dramatically due to advances in diagnostic technologies and the development of new therapies and medications. In response to these increased costs, which soon began spiraling out of control, a new third party payment system known as *managed care* was devised. The primary goal of managed care was to control costs by redistributing the financial risk involved in paying for healthcare.

Managed care can take a variety of forms. It is perhaps best to think of the managed care system as encompassing a continuum that moves from least structured—*managed indemnity plan*—to most structured—*Health Maintenance Organization* (or *HMO*). The different types of managed care plans may be described as follows:

1. *Managed Indemnity Plans* provide limited management of healthcare that is still paid for on a fee-for-service basis. These plans often employ utilization review strategies that may determine medical necessity prior to, for example, authorizing payment for hospital admission.

2. *Preferred Provider Organizations (PPOs)* are usually offered as one option in an insurance plan. PPO participants receive a comprehensive package of healthcare benefits as long as they receive care from healthcare professionals who are within the PPO's *preferred provider network*. Such healthcare professionals typically have entered into a contract with the PPO, stating that they will provide their services to PPO members for a reduced fee. This agreement is commonly entered into in exchange for an increased volume of patients. Patients can still elect to receive care from healthcare professionals who are outside this network but, if they do so, will be required to pay more of the costs themselves.

3. *Point of Service (POS) Plans* have been developed by managed care organizations as a means of offering enrolled persons a greater selection of physicians. Unlike the traditional HMO (see below), the POS plan may allow members to see a physician who is outside of the network, though they would face a higher premium, higher co-payment, higher deductible, or all three if they chose to do so.

4. *Health Maintenance Organizations (HMOs)* designate where and from whom members must, if they are to be covered, receive all of their healthcare services, as well as what types of medications may be covered. HMOs are able to reduce costs by contracting with, or owning, all of the entities involved in the provision

of healthcare that are covered by the HMO. Participants and/or employers usually pay lower premiums and lower co-pays in exchange for these reduced costs. Traditional HMOs use primary care providers (usually pediatricians, family practitioners, and internal medicine physicians) as so called "gate-keepers" to coordinate patient care. Such a mechanism requires that all referrals to specialty physicians be authorized by a patient's primary care doctor. Although patients are always free to visit any doctor they choose, their insurance will not pay anything for those visits unless they have been authorized in advance by their primary care physician.

Within this continuum of managed care options, the manner in which physicians or hospitals are reimbursed for the care they deliver varies greatly. Three primary forms of compensation are utilized. The first is a *discounted fee-for-service*. In this model, physicians or hospitals offer discounted fees to the HMO in exchange for increased patient volume. The second approach is *capitation*. With capitation, a predetermined amount of money (calculated as a certain amount per insured person per month) is paid to healthcare professionals to finance the care they will administer over a certain time period. In this type of system, the physician or hospital assumes some financial risk in delivering care because the amount of payment is not determined by the amount of services rendered. If the cost of services provided to those who are insured exceeds the amount of the negotiated payments, the hospital or physician will not receive compensation for the difference. If, on the other hand, surplus funds remain after all services have been provided, the physician or hospital will receive extra income. A third system relies on *re-insurance* and *stop loss pools,* which are often associated with insurance premiums that are reserved for the care of very ill (and therefore very costly) patients. Caring for a child with multiple handicaps, for example, may be so expensive and time-consuming that the physician actually loses money. In such cases, re-insurance or stop loss pools may be used to limit the degree to which a given healthcare professional is at financial risk, thereby allowing him or her to continue providing care. Once a certain amount of money has been lost on caring for a given patient, these mechanisms also may provide compensation and thereby limit ongoing losses. Finally, healthcare professionals who work within a capitated managed care system may receive payment (in the form of a salary) as employees of an HMO or may receive compensation through direct capitation.

Healthcare professionals who are reimbursed through any of the above models may be confronted with numerous ethical questions, especially when any of these arrangements are modified via bonuses or *withholds.* Withholds refer to the retaining by managed care organizations of a certain percentage of fees or salaries until year-end so that funds will be available to pay for any unanticipated surplus costs (e.g., re-insurance or stop loss pools). The assumption is that healthcare professionals with a vested interest in saving money on healthcare delivery may be more careful gatekeepers and only authorize "medically necessary" care. Such a system may indeed prompt some healthcare professionals to administer only this type of care; others, though, may be tempted to withhold care that a patient truly needs. The awarding of bonuses for the "most efficient" healthcare professionals may similarly cause some physicians to provide only needed care, but influence others to withhold care that is medically indicated. Such a system may also encourage doctors to see and treat only patients with less complicated healthcare problems who are less costly to manage.

29. Is managed care ethical?

In determining what's best for a patient, a physician's traditional focus has been exclusively on patient needs—not cost issues. But the development of new healthcare technologies and therapies has proven to be extremely expensive, and some people have complained that the co-mingling of cost containment and clinical judgment is eroding the medical profession's ideals. Managed care organizations (MCOs) come, however, in a variety of forms and raise different ethical issues. (See the answer to question 28 for an explanation of specific types of MCOs referred to below.)

Some MCOs, for example, are structured such that there is an incentive for physicians *not* to provide care. In this type of organization, e.g., a *capitation* system, a physician is paid a set fee for providing all the care a patient will need over a given period of time (such as one month). In such a system, the physician receives the same amount of money regardless of whether his patient has complicated conditions and is seen many times or has no problems and is never seen at all. This financial system completely separates the amount of payment from the type and frequency of care rendered, thereby placing physicians in a potential conflict of interest between their financial gain and the good of their patients. Under capitation models of payment, physicians assume some of the financial risk that may be involved in taking care of patients who have medically complex conditions and may require more visits or more expensive care; on the other hand, physicians may benefit financially by providing efficient care, only "medically necessary" care, or even less care than is needed.

Other MCOs attempt to manage healthcare costs by contracting with a group of physicians to provide care for a large number of patients. In exchange, physicians who are members of the managed care organization offer discounted fees for service. In this situation, the physician group stands to gain financially by increasing their patient volume, and the MCO gains financially by purchasing care for their members at a discounted rate.

Physicians who are salaried employees of a company receive compensation via another method of payment. As salaried employees they have no financial incentive to withhold care, but they also have no direct financial incentive to always provide all of the care that might be needed, causing some MCOs to have concerns about care delivery. This can be contrasted with the old *fee-for-service* model, where physicians had a financial incentive to provide *more* care than was necessary because they would receive additional compensation (even though excessive care could also pose a health risk to the patient). In other words, while managed care reimbursement systems have removed the latter unethical incentive, MCOs that continue to offer financial incentives and disincentives create other ethical conflicts for physicians. As explained near the end of the previous question, the conflicts can be multiplied when physician payment is modified by bonuses or withholds.

No matter what form of reimbursement is used, ethical conflicts can arise. It's important, therefore, that physicians adhere to sound ethical principles regarding financial matters. Physicians should see their primary goal as the good of patients, not their own financial gain. When healthcare professionals take this stance, they will be better able to resist patient demands for unneeded services or treatments (thus avoiding the excessive spending of fee-for-service models) as well as to resist temptations to improve either their own or their organization's profit at the patient's expense (thereby avoiding the potentially inadequate spending of managed care alternatives).

30. Is the healthcare industry like a business where the bottom line is profit?

Many people have become concerned that the healthcare industry is increasingly being run as if it were just another business. Indeed, the provision of healthcare has become based more and more on a business model: doctors and nurses are called "providers," patients are called "clients" or "customers," and healthcare itself is viewed as a "commodity." These developments are of concern because the healthcare profession should be about much more than simply exchanging services and materials for financial compensation.

Healthcare should not be viewed like other businesses for several reasons. First, patients usually seek professional healthcare when they are in a vulnerable state, sometimes in extreme need. If adequate care is not received, very serious consequences may result. This unique aspect of healthcare can be understood better if we contrast healthcare organizations with, for example, entertainment businesses. Everyone needs adequate healthcare, both to prevent illness and to bring healing when needed. By contrast, entertainment adds much to life, but those who can't afford it can still manage without this luxury. They may even be able to create their own entertainment for little or no cost. While people can likewise do much on their own to maximize their health, they are likely to require professional help at some point. Debate then arises over whether people have a right to healthcare, and, if so, what exactly this right entails (see the answer to question 18). Not debated, however, is that people need access to good healthcare, as they do to education, sanitation, protection, and a basic level of food and water. Healthcare is not subject to normal economic trade-offs; it's not something that people can go without in order to obtain more of other things they desire. Considering healthcare to be expendable in this way is tantamount to considering people to be expendable, and the resulting risks to human dignity are great.

While some people might argue that all businesses should place a higher priority on serving customers than on earning profits, most people acknowledge that profit is actually the bottom line for many businesses. A number of professions, though, including the healthcare profession, have traditionally not seen themselves as primarily profit-driven. Healthcare professionals should regard caring for people as their highest goal. Therefore, decisions will sometimes be made that are not in the best financial interests of the individual healthcare professional, clinic, or organization. Those who place a greater value on their mission to provide healthcare than on their profit margin may sometimes see diminished income and will likely give much of their earnings away in order to serve others. They may establish clinics and offer services in areas where people may not be able to pay much or at all. They may also volunteer their time to care for poor and needy persons.

Although the desire to serve in such a manner is indeed praiseworthy, those who take this approach could find themselves out of business if they spend more than they earn or receive in donations. Indeed, some non-profit healthcare organizations have avoided operating like a business to such an extent that they have not remained viable. A physician or nurse who offers care without ever earning any income will, in most cases, not be able to provide care for very long. Acquiring and using good business skills can be seen as a means for Christian healthcare professionals to exercise wise stewardship of the resources and opportunities that God provides for caring for others. Christian professionals would, nevertheless, do well to keep in view the examples of many great Christian men and women who have given sacrificially, depending upon God to provide—and He always has.

Emphasizing the *care* in healthcare should remind those interested in entering this field that it's not so much a profitable career as a calling. The many years of training, the long nights, and the tragic situations regularly encountered all call for people who are motivated to care sacrificially for others, not merely driven by the prospect of financial gain. We can be thankful that many Christians have entered the healthcare field because they sense a calling to serve, viewing healthcare as a way to exercise their God-given abilities to extend compassion and mercy to those in need.

Christians also play an important role in calling their professions to the highest ethical standards: those given by God. While Christian healthcare professionals do this regularly with regard to issues of life and death, they should be just as vigorous in applying God's standards to the financial decisions made at their healthcare organizations—thereby preventing profit from becoming the bottom line.

31. Should Christians consider funding healthcare through the Church?

Throughout the history of the Church, Christians have been actively involved in healthcare. Current hospital networks with names like *St. Joseph's* and *Methodist* signify that the Church has long played a significant role, while third-party health insurance (under which the patient is not solely responsible for covering healthcare costs) and government-based programs such as Medicaid and Medicare are relatively recent developments.

Church-based hospitals have throughout history provided

care for many patients who were unable to pay. Due to the increased costs of medical care and the decreased financial margin of many faith-based healthcare systems, their ability to cover the costs of caring for the poor has radically diminished. In addition, the rise of government payment for medical care through Medicare and Medicaid has changed the way that many faith-based clinics and hospital systems approach charity care. They will often now employ a social worker, who will pursue payment from Medicaid or Medicare.

Perhaps a better way to state the question here, then, is to ask how the Church should respond to the medical needs of the community. Are there new paradigms or ways of approaching the delivery of healthcare? The Church is currently addressing healthcare needs through a variety of methods. First, some denominations have developed their own health insurance companies. One example is *Mennonite Mutual Aid,* which offers decreased premiums since most Mennonites are in a low risk group because they do not smoke or drink alcohol. In addition, because fewer healthcare claims are submitted to this company, the company can choose to use any additional money to cover the costs of care incurred by particularly needy patients.

Second, many Catholic healthcare systems, which have traditionally used their funds to finance everything from hospitals to mobile healthcare vans, have begun to look at ways to leverage their extensive assets in order to provide more accessible or affordable care for those who are needy. The *Daughters of Charity,* for example, is a Catholic order that focuses on providing increased healthcare to poor persons by raising funds through thrift store profits and entering into joint medical business ventures.

Third, some within the Church are exploring other new paradigms. *Physicians Quality Healthcare* in Chicago,

Illinois, is a company actively involved in starting church-based health clinics through the *Jericho Road Foundation.* Setting clinics within churches allows for the provision of healthcare that many in the inner city lack and does so within a framework that allows for ministering to the whole person. Another novel approach is the *Christian Brotherhood Newsletter,* which was formed to facilitate the bearing of burdens between believers, based on Galatians 6:2. Members of the Brotherhood send a sum of approximately $150 per month to a fellow member who has significant outstanding medical expenses (such as those a patient would incur with hospitalization). Skilled persons within the Christian Brotherhood assist members in re-negotiating large medical bills from hospitalizations, frequently reducing the bill to Medicare rates (which are often 50 percent of the original bill). Since the amount of money sent to a Brotherhood member each month is usually less than that of a typical insurance premium, members are often able to save enough funds to take care of their day-to-day medical bills. In addition, patients who can pay cash for their medical expenses are frequently able to negotiate a significant reduction in routine fees due to saving their physicians the hassle and expense of dealing with insurance companies.

Christians can influence the amount of their healthcare expenses in two ways. First, the majority of one's healthcare costs are incurred in the final months of life, often in an attempt to prolong an inevitable death. Christians know that they will go to heaven after they die and, therefore, do not need to fear death. They may thus often choose to forego costly medical interventions that are not likely to significantly postpone death and thereby save a considerable amount of money. (See the *End of Life Decisions* booklet in this series for a full treatment of this complex area.) Such money may then be used to provide healthcare for those who are needy. Second, Christians, who have been commanded to regard their body as the "temple of God" (1 Cor. 3:16–17), have the responsibility to exercise preventive care (e.g., exercising regularly, maintaining a healthy weight, and not smoking). Christians should therefore be able to use the money saved on healthcare to benefit those in need.

If the Church is to follow Christ's example, it will unquestionably be involved in the provision and funding of healthcare. The real question concerns what methods it will choose for doing so. Although the above possibilities are by no means exhaustive, they may be helpful in equipping Christians to meet the healthcare needs of poor and underserved people and may stimulate further creative thinking on this issue.

Conclusion

Rapidly advancing technology has spawned medical research and related treatment options unheard of a generation ago. These newly developed medical technologies have not only made a bewildering array of treatment options and "improvement" interventions more available to patients, they have also come with the price of increased legal liability and economic expense. With the weakening of the traditional doctor-patient relationship, an increasing burden is placed on you as a patient to navigate the choppy ethical and economic waters of healthcare today.

Increasingly, people are turning to the Internet to get the information they need. While that can be a source of useful information, an Internet site can also be sprinkled with misinformation due to lack of careful review, or include a bias that comes from product or service marketing on that site. Internet sites can also have the same limitations as healthcare professionals—they can be guided by ethical values and quasi-religious beliefs that are very different from your own but in ways you do not recognize. So be proactive and discerning in your approach to gathering healthcare advice.

Knowing that the information you will obtain, the decisions you will make, and the care you will receive are filled with ethical considerations, do all you can to be faithful to God as you pursue them. As you trust in God's goodness, the Great Physician will provide for you far beyond what healthcare at its best can provide, so you do not need to be fearful in the face of today's healthcare challenges.

Using all of the counsel and people God has provided to help you make wise decisions is an important way to demonstrate your trust in God's provision.

Appendix:
Hippocratic Oath

I swear by Apollo the healer, by Aesculapius, by Health and all the powers of healing, and call to witness all the gods and goddesses that I may keep this Oath and Promise to the best of my ability and judgment.

I will pay the same respect to my master in the Science as to my parents and share my life with him and pay all my debts to him. I will regard his sons as my brothers and teach them the Science, if they desire to learn it, without fee or contract. I will hand on precepts, lectures, and all other learning to my sons, to those of my master and to those pupils duly apprenticed and sworn, and to none other.

I will use my power to help the sick to the best of my ability and judgment; I will abstain from harming or wrongdoing any man by it.

I will not give a fatal draught to anyone if I am asked, nor will I suggest any such thing. Neither will I give a woman means to procure an abortion.

I will be chaste and religious in my life and in my practice. I will not cut, even for the stone, but I will leave such procedures to the practitioners of that craft.

Whenever I go into a house, I will go to help the sick and never with the intention of doing harm or injury. I will not abuse my position to indulge in sexual contacts with the bodies of women or of men, whether they be freemen or slaves.

Whatever I see or hear, professionally or privately, which ought not to be divulged, I will keep secret and tell no one.

If, therefore, I observe this Oath and do not violate it, may I prosper both in my life and in my profession, earning good repute among all men for all time. If I transgress and forswear this Oath, may my lot be otherwise.

J. Chadwick and W. N. Mann, translator. *Hippocratic Writings*. New York: Penguin, 1950; http://www.medexplorer.com/content.dbm?Template=hippocratic.dbm (accessed March 17, 2004).

Recommended Resources

Cameron, Nigel M. de S. *The New Medicine: Life and Death After Hippocrates.* New ed. Chicago and London: Bioethics Press, LLC, 2001.

Kilner, John F., and C. Ben Mitchell. *Does God Need Our Help? Cloning, Assisted Suicide, & Other Challenges in Bioethics.* Wheaton, Ill.: Tyndale House, 2003.

Kilner, John F. *The Changing Face of Healthcare: A Christian Appraisal of Managed Care, Resource Allocation, and Patient-Caregiver Relationships.* Grand Rapids: Eerdmans, 1998.

May, William F. *The Physician's Covenant.* Philadelphia: Westminster/John Knox, 1983.

Orr, Robert D. *Medical Ethics: A Primer for Students.* Bristol, Tenn.: Paul Tournier Institute, 2000.

Pellegrino, Edmund D. *The Christian Virtues in Medical Practice.* Washington, D.C.: Georgetown University Press, 1996.

Endnotes

1. For an in-depth treatment of the Hippocratic Oath, we recommend that readers consult Nigel M. de S. Cameron, *The New Medicine: Life and Death After Hippocrates,* new ed. (Chicago and London: Bioethics Press, LLC, 2001).

2. See R. D. Orr et al., "Use of the Hippocratic Oath: A Review of Twentieth Century Practice and a Content Analysis of Oaths Administered in Medical Schools in the U.S. and Canada in 1993," *Journal of Clinical Ethics* 8, no. 4 (1997): 377–88.

3. David B. Larson and Susan S. Larson, *The Forgotten Factor in Physical and Mental Health: What Does the Research Show?* (Rockville, Md.: National Institute for Healthcare Research, 1994); and Dale Matthews, *The Faith Factor* (New York: Viking, 1998).

4. Harold G. Koenig, Michael E. McCullough, and David B. Larson, *Handbook of Religion and Health* (New York: Oxford University Press, 2001).

5. John W. Ehman, Barbara B. Ott, Thomas H. Short, Ralph C. Ciampa, and John Hansen-Flaschen, "Do Patients Want Physicians to Inquire About Their Spiritual or Religious Beliefs if They Become Gravely Ill?" *Archives of Internal Medicine* 159 (August 1999): 1803–6.

6. Not every state has adopted the so-called "Tarasoff rule," derived from the California case Tarasoff vs. Regents of University of California. 551 P. 2d 334 (Cal. 1976). In that case, the California Supreme Court held that a psychotherapist could be held liable for failing to exercise reasonable care to protect a third party when the therapist knows or should know that

her patient presents a serious danger of violence to another. It is not certain that the duty applies to physicians who are not in a therapeutic relationship with the patient. The duty to warn is imposed by state law; physicians are, therefore, advised to consult the laws of their own state.

7. "Personal Representatives," 3 April 2003, available at http://www.hhs.gov/ocr/hipaa/guidelines/personalrepresentatives.pdf (accessed 12 April 2004).

8. M. A. McCabe et al., "Implications of the Patient Self-Determination Act: Guidelines for Involving Adolescents in Medical Decision-Making," *Journal of Adolescent Health* 19, no. 5 (November 1996): 319–24.

9. See Nigel M. de S. Cameron, "Bioethics and the Challenge of a Post-Consensus Society," and David B. Fletcher's response, *Ethics and Medicine* 11, no. 1 (spring 1995): 1–12; K. Danner Clouser and Bernard A. Gert, "Critique of Principlism," *Journal of Medicine and Philosophy* 15, no. 2 (April 1990): 219–36; Richard A. McCormick, "Bioethics: A Moral Vacuum?" *America* 180, no. 15 (May 1999): 8–12; and David B. Fletcher, "The Ethics of Bioethics," *Dignity* 7, no. 2 (summer 2001): 3, 8. These matters are also addressed in the following footnote.

10. For example, Steve Wilkens, *Beyond Bumper Sticker Ethics* (Downers Grove, Ill.: InterVarsity, 1995). Also, John F. Kilner and C. Ben Mitchell, *Does God Need Our Help? Cloning, Assisted Suicide, and Other Challenges in Bioethics* (Wheaton, Ill.: Tyndale, 2003).

11. June Forkner-Dunn, "Internet-based Patient Self-care: The Next Generation of Healthcare Delivery," *Journal of Medical Internet Research* 5, no. 2 (2003): e8 (accessed at http://www.jmir.org/2003/2/e8/ on 7 August 2003).

12. Gretchen K. Berland et al., "Health Information on the Internet," *JAMA* 285 (2001): 2612–21.

13. Adapted from a story in: Steve Chalke, *He Never Said . . . : Discover the Real Message of Jesus* (London: Hodder and Stoughton, 2000), 113.

14. R. L. Berger, "Nazi Science: The Dachau Hypothermia Experiments," *The New England Journal of Medicine* 322, no. 20 (1990): 1435–40.

15. See www.stemcellresearch.org.

16. George W. Bush, "Remarks by the President on Stem Cell Research," available at http://www.whitehouse.gov/news/releases/2001/08/20010809-2.html (accessed 29 August 2003).

17. Linda K. Bevington, "Federally Funding Embryonic Stem Cell Research: Bush and Beyond," *Dignity* newsletter, fall 2001 (Bannockburn, Ill.: Center for Bioethics and Human Dignity), available at www.cbhd.org (accessed 20 October 2002).

18. See www.snowflakes.org.

19. Robert Orr, "Addressing Issues of Moral Complicity: When? Where? Why? and Other Questions," *Dignity* 9, no. 2 (spring 2003): 1, 5.